Advance Praise for

Healthy Happy sexy

"Ayurveda originated, in part, to address the disorders and ease the discomfort of a populous grown increasingly distant from the intimate practical knowledge of, and proximity to nature's cycles, seasons, and wisdom. Katie Silcox empathizes with these city and worldly dwellers, and shares simple, light-hearted, possibly life-changing perspectives and techniques that hail from the time-tested sisters in Indian sciences: Ayurveda and yoga."

—**Dr. Claudia Welch**, author of *Balance Your Hormones, Balance Your Life*

"Katie Silcox has written a practical, spicy, and highly readable manual for creating a workable Ayurvedic lifestyle. She makes this ancient traditional approach to health completely accessible—and in the process, inspires us to revolutionize our health by following the principles she outlines. Carefully researched and irradiated by Katie's own years of practice, this is a book to keep by your side for guidance through all the seasons of your life. I highly Recommend *Healthy Happy Sexy*—not least for the insights Katie offers on what it means to practice with the authenticity and radical self-honesty that real health and well being require!"

—**Sally Kempton**, world-renowned spiritual teacher, and author of
Awakening Shakti and *Meditation for the Love of It*

"Katie Silcox leads the next generation of thought leaders—helping people live healthier, happier, and more fulfilling lives. The fact that she can deliver what she has to say with so much clarity, humor, caring, and yes, sexiness is a gift, because it means that more and more of us will continue to be drawn to listen and thus, benefit from the ancient wisdom she so expertly conveys."

—**Rob Stryker**, pre-eminent yoga and meditation teacher, and author of
the bestseller *The Four Desires*

"Katie Silcox, you are the Carrie Bradshaw of the yoga and Ayurveda movement
in the United States."

—**Meredith Hogan**, voted Cincinnati's Best Yoga Teacher 2011

"Katie Silcox's voice is strong, clear, nourishing and empowering. *Healthy Happy Sexy* is a contemporary yogini's book of ancient secrets and profound knowledge of our body, spirit and soul. Katie masterfully presents the philosophy and practices of Ayurveda with her own wisdom and experience. She shows how we can create our own journey into wellness and embrace our inherent sexual and creative power. Her book is an open–hearted and soulful invitation to align our natural rhythm with Mother Earth so that we too may reap the benefits of a balanced and harmonious life. Katie's wise and witty guidance inspires us to make empowered choices about wellness so we can live a life of juicy freedom. This beautiful and inspiring book is for any woman who wants to come into alignment with herself and the Divine."

—**Laura Amazzone**, author of *Goddess Durga* and *Sacred Female Power*

"Katie Silcox's book, and indeed her life, is filled with refreshingly real, flowingly connected, and valuably accessible moments of Kala-Deshi-Patra, making her work more potentially 'Authentic Ayurveda' than the literally outdated Victorian attitudes that have attenuated Ayurveda's blossoming for many decades now. Katie's book feeds her readers, no doubt, but more importantly in many ways, it also nourishes the Ayurvedic tradition itself. By giving it a new license, and thus a new life, she sustains the perennial wisdom of this grand 'Science of Life.'"

—**Prashanti de Jager, MS**, founder of Organic India and The Pacific Center for Ayurveda, author of *Turmeric: The Ayurvedic Spice of Life*

"*Happy Healthy Sexy* is a great introduction to the timeless wisdom of Ayurveda and is brought to life by Katie Silcox, one of a new generation of gifted writers. Intelligently written and witty, readers will be inspired to take greater care of their sacred self and bring the sacred into everyday life."

—**Dr. Marc Halpern**, president of the California College of Ayurveda and author of *Healing Your Life*

"Katie translates the self-help ancient system of Ayurveda for the modern woman who wants to be more healthy, happy, and sexy and achieve the goals of pleasure, prosperity, purpose, and freedom—living life to the fullest."

—**Sharon Gannon**, founder of Jivamukti Yoga

"Katie Silcox's enthusiasm for yoga, Ayurveda, and loving relationships radiates with heart-warmth on every page of *Healthy Happy Sexy*. This book is packed with loads of information from the deep well of Indic traditional knowledge, all conveyed with her great joy and love of life."

—**Stuart Sovatsky, PhD**, copresident of the Association for Transpersonal Psychology and author of *Advanced Spiritual Intimacy* and *Your Perfect Lips*

"Katie Silcox is a breath of fresh, feminine air. She has the innate ability to translate ancient teachings into modern language that is tangible, relatable, funny, and by the end of the book you feel as though you have been sharing secrets with your dearest friend. And, Katie is just that. She is a friend for all who seek to know more of their wonderful, juicy, and highest Self. This book is an amazing vehicle for those who are ready to begin a journey towards happiness and health. It is also a must-have reference for teachers and students who are passionate about the possibility of transformation, and of course, bringing sexy back."

—**Jessica Durivage-Kerridge**, founder of Where Is My Guru, writer, speaker, yoga teacher, and Divine Mama at www.whereismyguru.com

"I have complete trust in Katie. She is one of those very rare yoga teachers for whom the inner journey is both central and powerful. You get the sense when you are around her that she's been down this road before, that there's a deep wisdom about yoga and Ayurveda encoded into her system and she's waking up to it anew right in front of your eyes. She sparkles when she teaches and her path of ParaYoga shares unique secrets about breathing and posture found in no other tradition. If you are open to being transformed, visit her classes and enjoy the benefit of her soft touch and a wisdom that belies her years."

—**Eric Shaw**, founder of Prasana Yoga and Yoga Education Through Imagery

Student and Client Testimonials

"The first time I met Katie, my heart was simultaneously melted and set on fire by her teaching and presence. This woman has the rare gift of being able to pierce to the heart of a teaching and express it in a way that is not only clear and practical, but also dripping with aliveness, humor, and pure love. Katie is a walking, dancing, radiant embodiment of yoga. She is an Ayurvedic alchemist, a transformer of lives, and an awakener of magic. I am so grateful she has shown up in my life."

—**Seren Rubens**, yoga teacher, Nevada City, California

"Almost every woman I know fights the same battle, struggling to maintain a tenuous balance between what we want (everything) and what we feel we should have (nothing). Katie is a mind-bendingly good teacher, whose approach to healing is holistic, passionate, integrative, and enormously engaging and fun. The war is over! I've never felt more at home in my body and I'm convinced that joy is a vital part of health. Katie offers an almost bacchanalian celebration, inviting us to get on the 'goddess-schedule,' including herbs, unbridled laughter, singing, chanting, sharing, and sacred silence. Being with Katie is an invitation into the blessing of recognizing our whole selves—our delusions, as well as what is truly alive in our hearts. Thank you, thank you, thank you."

—**Sarah Norris**, writer, editor, and yoga teacher, Nashville, Tennessee

"I appreciate and adore Katie's ability to translate and provide the teachings of Tantra in an accessible and digestible way. I have been studying this material for two years and sitting and practicing with Katie for one week literally brought the teachings to life. I not only learn in a way that seeps into my pores but I experience the teachings when with her in a way that is powerful and impacting."

—**Kim Garrison Burriss**, psychotherapist, San Francisco, California

"Katie's words are direct and imbued with the love that she is. They reverberate through me, reminding me to come back to Presence. To come back to Love. I am so blessed to learn and experience tried and true Ayurvedic and Tantric methods for health and soul liberation from such a grounded, humble, driven, radiant soul, and adept on the spiritual path."

—**Rhani Lee Remedes**, rockstar, healer, and yoga teacher, San Francisco, California

"The most significant changes that I have experienced since this training have been around my personal practice, teaching practice, and the way I come to make choices, decisions and set goals for myself. I left feeling grounded, and well equipped with tools that would weave beautifully into an increasingly fulfilling experience of teaching, practice, and life back home."

—**Sylvie Anne Hotchkins,** yoga teacher, Montreal

Healthy
Happy
sexy

Healthy Happy Sexy

AYURVEDA WISDOM for MODERN WOMEN

Katie Silcox

ATRIA PAPERBACK
New York London Toronto Sydney New Delhi

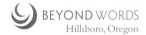
BEYOND WORDS
Hillsboro, Oregon

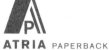

ATRIA PAPERBACK
A Division of Simon & Schuster, Inc.
1230 Avenue of the Americas
New York, NY 10020

BEYOND WORDS
20827 N.W. Cornell Road, Suite 500
Hillsboro, Oregon 97124-9808
503-531-8700 / 503-531-8773 fax
www.beyondword.com

Managing editor: Lindsay S. Brown
Editors: Emily Han, Gretchen Stelter
Copyeditor: Claire Rudy Foster
Proofreader: Linda M. Meyer
Design: Devon Smith
Composition: William H. Brunson Typography Services

First Atria Paperback/Beyond Words trade paperback edition January 2015

For more information about special discounts for bulk purchases, please contact Simon & Schuster Special Sales at 1-866-506-1949 or business@simonandschuster.com.

The Simon & Schuster Speakers Bureau can bring authors to your live event. For more information or to book an event, contact the Simon & Schuster Speakers Bureau at 1-866-248-3049 or visit our website at www.simonspeakers.com.

Manufactured in the United States of America

10 9 8 7 6 5 4 3

Library of Congress Cataloging-in-Publication Data

Silcox, Katie.
    Healthy happy sexy : ayurveda wisdom for modern women / Katie Silcox.
        pages   cm
    1. Women—Health and hygiene.   2. Medicine, Ayurvedic.   I. Title.
    RA778.S583   2015
    613′.04244—dc23

                                                                    2014024638

ISBN 978-1-58270-473-9
ISBN 978-1-4767-5738-4 (eBook)

The corporate mission of Beyond Words Publishing, Inc.: *Inspire to Integrity*

Dedication

To my first mama, Vera Jessee Silcox. And to Yogarupa Rod Stryker, who taught me about my Divine Mama.

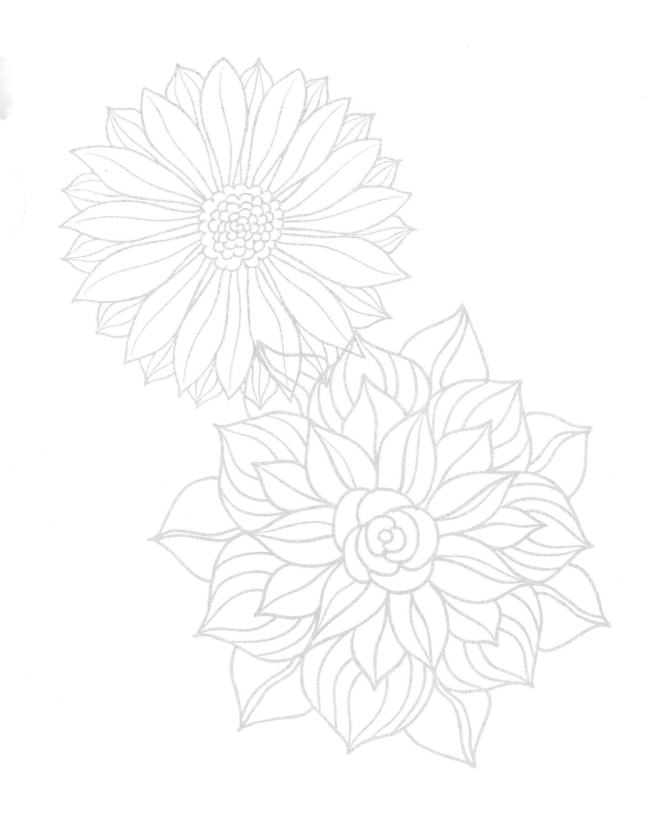

Contents

Part IV: Sexy

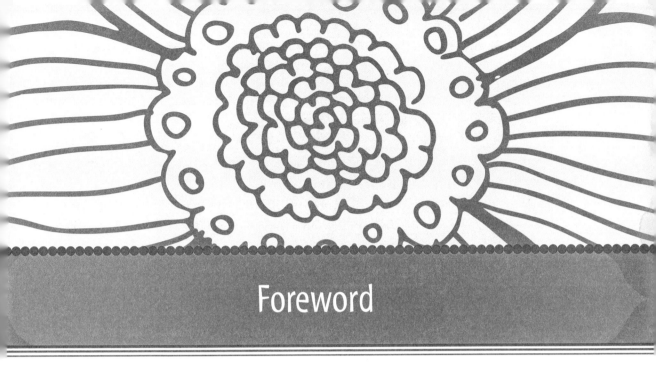

Foreword

This book has the potential to dramatically improve the quality of your life—hard to believe, particularly if you are unfamiliar with the world of Ayurveda and the extraordinary wisdom upon which it is based. It is hard to grasp all that it has to offer, in large part, because *Healthy Happy Sexy* is about accessing a kind of far-reaching health and well-being that is rarely discussed in Western culture. We don't see or hear about it on TV. Celebrities don't talk about it when promoting themselves or their health and beauty secrets. We weren't taught about Ayurveda in school, and few modern-day health professionals, even if they are experts in their chosen field, have a working knowledge of it. Therefore, this book is truly a gift: it speaks directly, practically, and with real insight into modern life and how we can achieve the life that all of us, in our hearts, deeply long for—a life that must include radi-

ant health, along with happiness and lasting fulfillment.

The truth is that while we may be living longer, we may not necessarily be living better. Despite all the technology we have at our fingertips, research shows that we are, on the whole, less happy and in many ways less healthy. Many of our most common ailments and diseases are now simply accepted as the price of getting older and living longer. We assume that not being able to sleep through the night is no big deal, if only because we don't know anyone else that does. Similarly, more and more of us don't have enough energy to get through our day (without dosing ourselves with caffeine or other stimulants). Too many of us—whether we are aware of it or not—live with persistent, low levels of anxiety, depression, or distress and weakened immune, digestive, or eliminative systems. Nearly all of

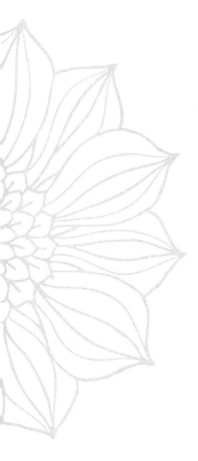

us remember less than we used to, find it hard to focus, and suffer from a decreased sex drive.

In the last decade or so, it seems that anxiety, sadness, and fatigue have become the new "normal." Of course, modern medicine and drug companies are at the ready with remedies to temporarily relieve our symptoms, and since we all want to feel our best—or at least manage our pain—we consume these modern prescriptions. In the process, we spend billions of dollars; meanwhile, what we truly seek—lasting happiness and radiant health and the sense that our lives are meaningful—isn't getting any closer.

It wasn't always like this. Think back. I am certain you can recall a sense of being so fully alive and feeling so good that the thought that you could feel better never occurred to you. Don't recall that feeling? What about your early childhood? For most of us, the early years of life provide a picture of real health—which is not the same as the absence of disease. Indeed, real health, as described by the ancient tradition of Ayurveda, borders on the sublime. It is a quality that is abundant in childhood, when we are filled with boundless enthusiasm, curiosity, and vitality. We were all once endlessly energetic and full of wonder, practically swimming in a world of possibility. There was magic in all you encountered and in your very being—so much so that you assumed it would never end. Oh yeah, and you slept like a baby. Remember that? If you are lucky, it lasted until you were thirty or so, and then it started to gradually fade. That was when responsibilities, stress, obligations, anxiety, aging, drinking, some unwise choices about your diet, heartache, and the basic wear and tear of a busy life began to accumulate. At some point, slowly, undetectably, things changed and the new you overshadowed the original, youthful you. You didn't actually change, but something that you once had in great supply was not as available. For most of us, even before the middle of our life is over, much of our initial endowment of resilience, joy, creativity, strength, inspiration, passion, and potential has become a memory.

Recovering these and reawakening to all the possibilities—and the gift of life itself—is the underlying intent of Ayurveda, and it is what this book is all about. Few systems dedicated to promoting health and well-being the world over can match the profound and comprehensive approach that you will find in these pages. Few, if any, can rightfully claim that their content has been improving human beings' quality of life for thousands of years—this one can. Most importantly, despite being rooted in ancient, time-tested wisdom, the practice of Ayurveda, as outlined in this book, could not be more relevant to you and your life today. You're dealing with very real challenges, while trying to not lose sight of your hopes and aspirations. In short, this book is an incredible resource for anyone interested in better health, more vitality, peace of mind, more capacity, freedom, joy, better sleep, and yes, even better sex. And therein is the main point of *Healthy Happy Sexy*. Despite its span of wonderful and detailed wisdom, its focus is simple: helping you have more of what you want, and less of what you don't.

I could not be more pleased that Katie Silcox—whom I have had the pleasure to know and teach for more than a decade and who so thoroughly understands and embodies this material—has brought her considerable talent to write a modern definitive primer on Ayurveda. Katie is passionate about the subject. She has seen it change her clients' bodies as well as their souls. In these pages, she speaks to you as a sister, friend, and kind and loving guide (with a sense of humor, no less) to lead you delightfully to the banquet of self-care that is Ayurveda. Through her expert guidance, you will learn how to recognize and nurture the unique attributes that make you who you are; you will learn about the simple choices you can make every day to honor the best of you and celebrate your life.

Having personally benefited from Ayurveda so richly and watched it contribute to the lives of countless others who I have taught and counseled, I am quite certain that as you apply the wisdom on these pages, you will soon begin to feel healthier and more inspired, radiant, and rested. And who doesn't want that? Nonetheless, I would invite you to stay mindful of the larger picture; the ultimate intention of Ayurveda is to provide you with more than just radiant health. Its ultimate aim is to help you ignite the full force of your spirit.

As you set out into the inspired and profound teachings in this book, you will soon discover Ayurveda to be a vast and complex body of knowledge—you might feel overwhelmed by how much there is to learn. As Katie suggests: "Don't be." It is neither essential nor necessary that you know all the contents of this (or any other) book about Ayurveda. This is not a book to study as much as it is a book to live by and, most importantly, to practice. Start wherever you are. Apply the things you find here that speak most loudly to you and your heart. You will be eternally thankful that you did.

Ayurveda is one of the greatest and most complete systems of self-care ever developed. It is designed to help you gain essential insight into yourself and to lead you to greater balance. As you become more balanced, your mind will become clearer and more focused, and as a result, the full force of your soul or spirit *will* fully shine. In the process, your life will take on greater meaning. You will see beauty, feel the magic of your childhood, and have an enduring sense that your life is truly a gift. You will discover spontaneity, as well as love. You will learn to care for yourself and the world in which you live. Thus, you will become most fully yourself—the very person that nature intended you to be. Without a doubt, applying what you learn from these pages will have a positive effect on you, those around you, and the world we all live in. Don't wait. Don't hesitate. Enjoy.

Rod Stryker
2014

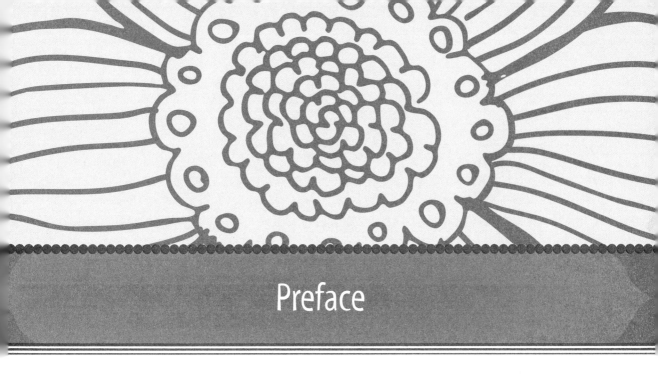

Preface

After years of schmoozing with zany technologists, government agents, Chicago stockbrokers, and a nearly endless parade of secretly sleepless coworkers, I decided that corporate America was slowly sucking away my soul. I had a hunger to know myself. I watched as people who had cash, cars, designer clothes, and power drowned their minds with alcohol, prescription drugs, and other pain-numbing tactics. It was more than my heart could bear.

I was also experiencing my own host of imbalances—almost unbearable anxiety, crash diets to get rid of late night dinner parties, addiction to caffeine to wake up, alcohol to relax after work, and cigarettes to take the edge off. One day my boss offered me a raise and a promotion—and I went home and cried. I felt like I was on a precipice, where rational choice (*duh, take the job*) was trumped by a little cry from my heart saying, "Save yourself."

You see, I wanted to live a purpose-driven life—something that all the money; beautiful, power-elite friends; and my understanding of the world at that time would never satisfy. I wanted to live a life of fullness—the kind of life that continually allowed my heart to open—whether it was breaking from sadness or bursting with awe. I wanted to live in integrity with my own version of God. I wanted to learn how to listen to my body. I wanted to smell grass and dirt, and learn about plants.

So, I turned down the job offer. Luckily, I had enough savings to spend some time really getting serious about loving and taking care of myself (something that was put to the wayside in my former life). I started practicing yoga and meditation every day. I studied health and

Ayurvedic Terms

Ayurvedic teachings were originally written in Sanskrit, but I have tried my best to use as little of this ancient language as possible. That said, there are many words in Sanskrit that are simply too beautiful to leave out. Some don't have an English equivalent and therefore are cool to learn. It's kind of like how Inuit people have hundreds of words for snow because of the complexity of their understanding. The ancients understood the body and the mind in depth. Moreover, Sanskrit words are more than just words; they are supercharged sounds that connect our senses to the original Seer Sages and Shamanic Mamas who lived and breathed this wonderful science. I hope you will enjoy learning some exotic new words. At the very least, you can slip them into your next cocktail party conversation.

wellness ravenously, reading everything I could get my hands on regarding herbs, energy work, Eastern philosophy, and Western ideas of how the mind and body were connected.

This passion led me to travel the world, studying with many great teachers to try to unlock the secret of balanced living. I saw Tibetan *amchis* in Ladakh heal people through absolute miracles and magic. I watched Sufis spin on the beaches of Goa. I witnessed MIT mathematicians weep at the beauty of golden ratio patterns in nature. I shared visions with shamans in Morocco. I learned about the subtle ways we store our emotions on our breath in Chennai, India. I meditated with plant spirits in Northern California. I studied with some of the East's and the West's most renowned teachers and healers of Ayurveda, Taoism, Tibetan and Indian Tantra, and yoga. And I practiced what they taught me.

Out of all my studies into mind-body health, it was yoga, and especially the self-care aspect of yoga called Ayurveda (the principle foundation for this book) that stuck out. I found these ancient practices for self-healing to be powerful, intuitive, and incredibly nurturing. What my body and soul needed was to be deeply loved—and Ayurveda offered that in spades. The more I worked with the principles of Ayurveda, the more my anxious heart calmed down. My body got simultaneously stronger and softer. I learned how to work with my emotions, learned a form of self-care that would feed and energize my body and teach me to become intimate with my sexuality in powerful new ways. Simply put, I started to feel truly at home in my own skin. The body that I had once criticized and disconnected from was now a temple to be honored and cared for. Today, I'm still learning; it's an ongoing journey. But I am deeply grateful for the answered prayer that is the wisdom of Ayurveda. I know it saved my life.

My first teacher of Ayurveda, an Indian yogi named A.G. Mohan, used to encourage us—avid students that we were—not to think we needed to eat Indian food or chant Indian mantras to be healthy and achieve enlightenment.

"It is simple," he would say. "Just eat what your grandmother cooked for you. Your body will be nourished by that. Worship the gods of your own ancestors. Your body and spirit will recognize them."

"But what if some of our grandmothers fed us corndogs and blue Slush Puppies from the 7-Eleven?" I protested (to myself).

Eventually I came to see that Ayurveda is not necessarily about what my actual grandmother would have fed me; it is about channeling my own inner grandma—make that the hippest, sassiest, most contented version of my grandma that I could imagine. I thought, *What if I channeled the combined wisdom of all of our grandmothers and great-grandmothers?* I could feel their wrinkled hands as they chopped onions for chicken soup to dose their grandchildren's colds. I felt the love and intuition that went into the preparation of a simple plant remedy. I anchored myself in the ancient wisdom of their laughter, stories, and healing.

My inner grandma was not just wise and wrinkled; she was also magically young and full of energy. She was not only loving, but also possessed the no-bullshit sense of a saucy, organic-garden-tending Michelle Obama. She could deliver a baby, bandage a wound, dance the samba or run off to Burning Man. When the stars aligned, my inner grandma could cook a mean bone-broth stew, lead a yoga class, and even release herself to the throes of killer multiple orgasms. In summer, she was sleek, like a deer covered in coconut oil. In fall, she was intuitively internal, wrapped in wool and meditating on the moon. In winter, she prepared for the coming rebirth, and in spring, she burst forth like a wanton orchid. My inner grandma was seasonally hip and irreverently spiritual. She was an impish goddess, completely aligned with the biggest grandma of all, Mother Nature. She was inside of me, roaring to be released—and she is inside of you as well. This is the force that Ayurveda enables us to reconnect with, and it is to that invincible Her inside each of you that I dedicate this book.

Today, I am blessed to be a senior teacher under the ParaYoga Sri Vidya lineage of Tantra, and have practiced this system for over a

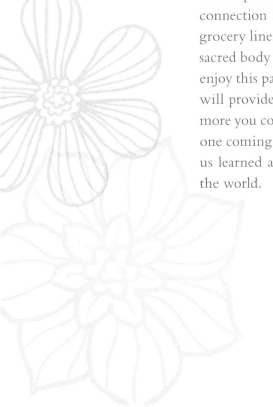

decade. I am lucky to say that during this time, I have had the same teacher and mentor—Yogarupa Rod Stryker, who is widely considered to be one of the preeminent yoga and meditation teachers in the United States. Under the guidance of yoga and Ayurveda's incredible system of self-empowerment, I have become an internationally traveling yoga teacher, writer, and founder of a Tantric yoga teacher training school. I also ended up graduating from one of the country's best Ayurveda schools and have become an Ayurvedic healer myself.

This book is an offering of what I've learned and lived thus far, particularly in the realm of Ayurveda. Ayurveda is a life science that understands that Mother Nature is the boss of us. When we learn her rhythms and tendencies, both inside ourselves and out in the world, we feel better. We have more energy. Our mind is calmer. Our vision is clearer. Our hearts are more open. I have now been a teacher of yoga and a practitioner of Ayurveda for over a decade, and I can attest to the power of this system to radically, yet gently, change your life.

May Ayurveda lead you, my sensual goddess, toward radical self-empowerment through the realization of a deep and intimate connection between the "out-there" world of relationships, traffic, grocery lines and crying babies, and the "in-here" world of your own sacred body and mind. Jump into this journey, and most importantly, enjoy this path toward health, radiance, and sexual vitality. This book will provide you with practical tools to help you get there. And the more you come back into balance, the more you are supporting everyone coming back into spiritual integrity with our planet. If enough of us learned and practiced Ayurvedic wisdom, we could even change the world.

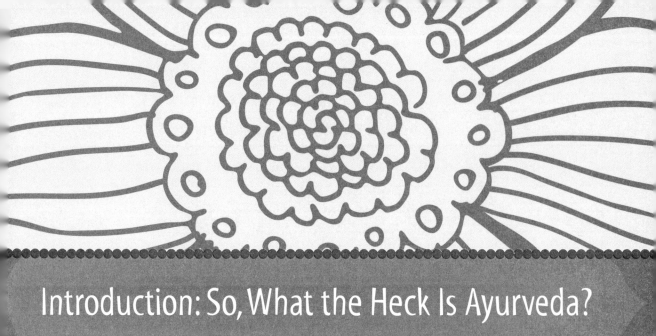

Introduction: So, What the Heck Is Ayurveda?

on't worry. The first time I tried to say the word Ayurveda, I too had to twist and contort my tongue. The word is pronounced AYE-YOUR-VAY-DA, with the accent on the VAY. The word comes from the combination of *ayur*, meaning life, and *veda*, meaning knowledge. So Ayurveda is literally "the knowledge of life," how to live life in the best possible way. It is a back-to-basics, natural approach to living—a complex mix of oral and written instruction, philosophy, mythology, spirituality, and scientific knowledge. It is highly evolved folk medicine and tradition— simple yet profound, mundane but magical.

Ayurveda is one of the four Upavedas, or secondary teachings, rooted in the oldest spiritual texts of ancient India, the Vedas. Widely considered to be humanity's most ancient healing science, these millennia-old texts address all aspects of healing and well-

being for both the body and mind. Much of this tradition of Ayurvedic medicine and philosophy was transmitted orally, from teacher to student. Today, we are blessed with several seminal texts that form the basis of classic Ayurvedic medicine and organize the principles of its philosophy. These texts and practices date back to somewhere between 450-1500 BCE and include the *Caraka Samhita*, *Sushruta Samhita*, *Ashtanga Hridayam*, *Ashtanga Samgraha*, *Madhava Nidanam*, and the *Sarangadhara Samhita*.[1]

Ayurveda originated in the early Indus Valley civilization, and eventually gained great prestige, spreading out all over India, Sri Lanka, and even into Tibet, China, and Nepal. In fact, it formed the basis for many forms of traditional medicine practiced in these countries in later years. Sadly, the colonization of India brought an abrupt end to Ayurveda's thriving. The colonists denounced Ayurveda as a backward, inferior folklore and replaced it with western medicine. Luckily, Ayurveda continued to be practiced beneath the radar of colonists in rural areas and in monasteries.[2] Today, it is undergoing a huge resurgence in India and North America as well as many other Western countries, as we look to combine the science and technology of traditional Western medicine with Ayurveda's holistic, preventative healing arts. Its renaissance is even more understandable here in the United States, as healthcare costs surge and many of us seek prevention as a means of empowerment, as well as beginning to look more toward nature-based healing.

Radical Self-Honesty and Awareness

Ayurveda is a philosophy and an approach to wellness that holds self-awareness as the essence and foundation of good health. Its long-revered teachings offer insights so simple yet so profound that you may have a hard time believing how powerful they are. And how do we align ourselves with this cosmic sweetness, according to Ayurveda? By learning how to live in accordance with the never-ending ebb and flow of the Big Mama herself: Mother Nature.

Ayurveda not only aligns us with the macrocosm of Big Mama, but it also helps us learn to dive deep inside the mini-universe of ourselves through self-observation and self-love. True self-seeing requires a willingness to look deeply at our own life challenges and areas of confusion. It asks us to ponder difficult questions like, "Where is my life lacking sweetness and nurturing to such an extent that I find myself reaching for bonbons late at night, snuggling up with a wine bottle, or calling up ex-boyfriends I had good reasons for leaving?" This type of inner-looking is vital because the more we understand the dark corners of our heart, the more our body and mind will naturally begin to align with the purity that is our true nature.

This path I will lead you down is not always easy. It requires radical self-honesty, compassion, contemplation, and regular meditation. (Yes, I said the M word. But don't worry; this book will make it easy for you to start meditating if you've never done it before.) This path also requires a shift in self-care and responsibility. A central tenet of Ayurveda is that the small choices we make every day can dramatically affect our health over time. We must accept ownership of and responsibility for our life circumstances. That means we have to own our late-night emotional eating, insomnia, undigested father issues, financial woes, and any other stuff that's keeping us stuck.

When we are truly honest and learn to digest our life circumstances, we take a giant step toward empowerment. How does this work? Ayurveda understands that our old, unhelpful patterns simply cannot be overcome without acceptance and compassion. Of course, we can't change all of our life circumstances, but we can adjust our reaction to them. It is this internal readjustment that eventually frees us from the suffering. The practices in this book will help you discover that you have a choice; you can become the author of your own story instead of the victim of it.

Using Ayurvedic principles of health and lifestyle will give us the tools for enjoying the healthiest, happiest, and sexiest life ever. We will go from being victims to being cocreators of what we really want—a fabulously healthy body, a calm mind, and a big ol' heart. Ayurveda gives us the unlimited potential to get all three, all by becoming more present, more aware, and more attuned to Mother Nature.

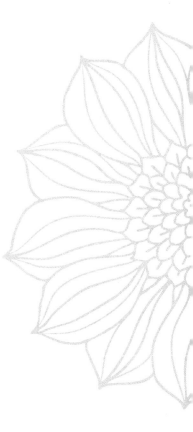

Mother Nature? What If I Live in New York?

I know it may seem challenging to think of aligning with the tides of Nature. Many of the women I know live in crowded cities and tight apartments. Or are go-getter mamas trucking their kids around town to endless extracurricular activities, battling busy highways, drinking supercharged double espresso macchiatos. All of us communicate in realtime on the information superhighway, texting instant messages to distant loved ones. It stands to reason that amid the speed and information overload of life in the modern world, we struggle with creating balance as natural beings, as women. If you are a radiance-seeking, spirit-minded, time-constrained woman, this book is for you.

I used to be exactly that kind of woman. I lived in the hustle and bustle of the San Francisco Bay Area, and I felt crummy a lot of the time. The only things that really helped me get balanced came from Ayurveda. When I started studying its teachings, I discovered that the women of centuries past were not as disconnected from their innate healing capacities as women of today. They used ancient tools and techniques for self-care and nourishment, and these very same tools can make life in today's labyrinth of the hectic Western world much easier. Much calmer. Much happier. And most importantly, these tools can lead us to a feeling of deep satisfaction within the complex tapestry of our everyday life.

So, to all of you urban and suburban women reading this, there is hope for us. The beauty of Ayurveda is that it was as relevant to a woman of ancient India (who had plenty of time to lather her nipples in oil steeped in frankincense, chew on fenugreek seeds, and anoint her body in preparation for her lover) as it is to the modern-day lady (who knows she's doing really well if she can manage to shave her legs for her lover). It is about cultivating the ability to empower yourself to lead a healthy, balanced life that doesn't sacrifice our natural sensual pleasures.

How to Use This Book— Avoiding Ayurveda Overwhelm

Remember that it will not be helpful to try to implement all of this book tomorrow. Begin slowly. I recommend reading the book from the beginning to learn the beauty and practicality of the Ayurveda philosophy, and then move onward into the 3 main parts of the book: Healthy, Happy, and Sexy. Then, implement 1–2 things that you can really commit to for the next few weeks. After you feel comfortable with those, pick up another few recommendations. Over time, these suggestions will become natural and part of your everyday life. Keep in mind that Ayurveda is vast, and it will take time to fully grasp its reach. Settle for learning it a piece at a time. Read the ideas in this book slowly and let them sink into your consciousness.

After you have read through the book, put it in your kitchen, or beside your bathtub or bed—anywhere you need advice, inspiration, or a gentle reminder. I also suggest having a journal by your side while working with this book. This will help you document your experience, keeping you connected to your own inner voice. I offer some reflections and action steps at the end of each chapter for cultivating more intimacy with your Ayurveda experience and, most importantly, yourself.

This journey you're about to embark upon will be one of the most rewarding of your life, but remember to take it one step at a time—and to take it easy on yourself. You picked up this book, most likely, because you want to have more nature in your life, more love, more happiness, and more self-acceptance. None of us got to where we are today—whether we're thrilled with life or struggling a little—overnight. So keep your journal beside you, keep an open mind, and just keep on the path. We'll get there together as you start your journey toward being healthy, happy, and sexy.

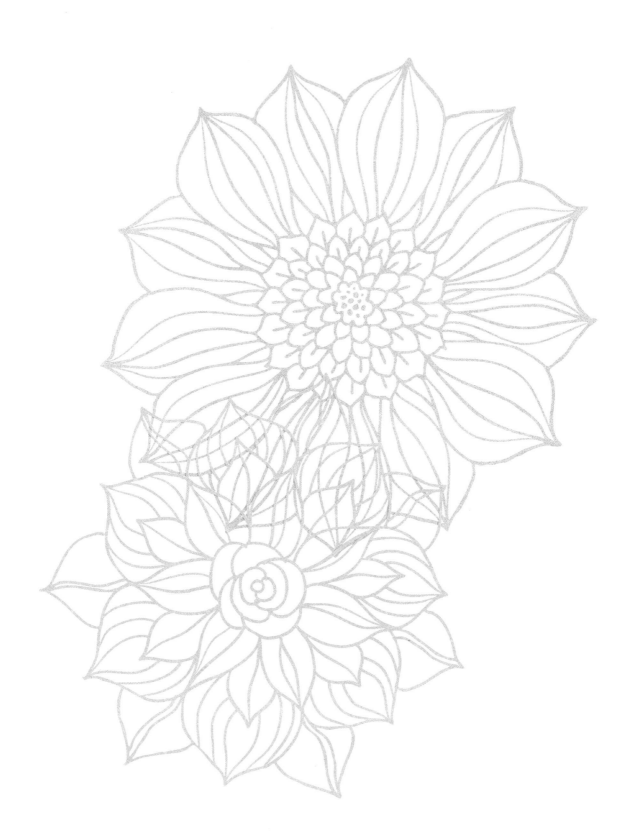

Part I

Philosophy

*B*efore we dive into the breadth of rituals, routines, and recommendations that Ayurveda provides, we're going to back things up just a bit and give you an idea about where this all came from. Ayurveda is a complex and ancient system of well-being, and just as Western medicine is based on biology and other sciences that can take a lifetime to understand, Ayurveda has many foundational concepts and tenets that you can explore and deepen your understanding of, for years and years.

For our purposes, there are some basic principles that we'll start with, so you have a clearer grasp of Ayurveda's view of the universe—both macro and micro—and our relationship to it and each other. These basic tenets of Ayurveda are really a jumping off point both for introducing Ayurvedic ideas into your everyday life and for further study, should you wish to do so, of the deeper philosophies of Ayurveda.

If you have a yoga practice, you can also look at this Ayurvedic foundation as a way to deepen that practice. The mat-based poses many of us would refer to as "yoga" encompass just the tip of the iceberg that is the broader Vedic tradition. A part of this is Ayurveda, yoga's forgotten but incredibly important sister science.

Think of yoga and Ayurveda as two interrelated branches of the same massive tree of Vedic knowledge, each playing its own role in your journey toward health, happiness, and vitality. While yoga typically deals with the use of techniques such as *asana* (postures), *mantras* (sacred transformational sounds), and *pranayama* (the management of energy), Ayurveda deals with reducing disease and healing the body and mind.

Yoga supports your health; living an Ayurvedic lifestyle, like the one you will learn in this book, supports your spiritual journey. While yoga supports healing, it is the ancient art of Ayurveda that teaches us how to heal.

My Own Ayurveda Philosophy Journey

I first heard Ayurveda philosophy from the lips of two master yoga teachers in India—A.G. and his wife Indra Mohan. I was sitting on the floor of their home in South India. A.G. spoke of the Universe being comprised of five essential elements (we will get to them soon). And I remember thinking, *What is this beautiful old man talking about?* It seemed "out there." I honestly wondered if what he was teaching me would *ever* have an application in my life as a technology-loving, microwave-using, hamburger-eating, at-times-cross Western woman. But there he sat, so handsome and young looking for an older man! He was healthy. He radiated a glowing kindness. And he was clearly happy. I daresay that his beautiful wife Indra was downright sexy in her sixties!

But the philosophy still felt farfetched to me at that time. Perhaps the loving knowingness coming from A.G. and Indra Mohan was enough to encourage me to trust in Ayurveda. I started reading books on the topic. I began to meditate more. I applied the oils they suggested to my body. I started breathing in a calmer way. I practiced a slower-moving form of yoga. I ate more warm, cooked foods. I spent more time in nature, and in silence.

Today, Ayurveda feels as real to me as a hug from my sister. It lives in my body, and I am constantly humbled to see these principles alive in Mama Nature. I say this to you because I want you to take your time with the philosophical concepts in this book. With a little effort on the practical end, you will start to see how these ancient truths can become real for you.

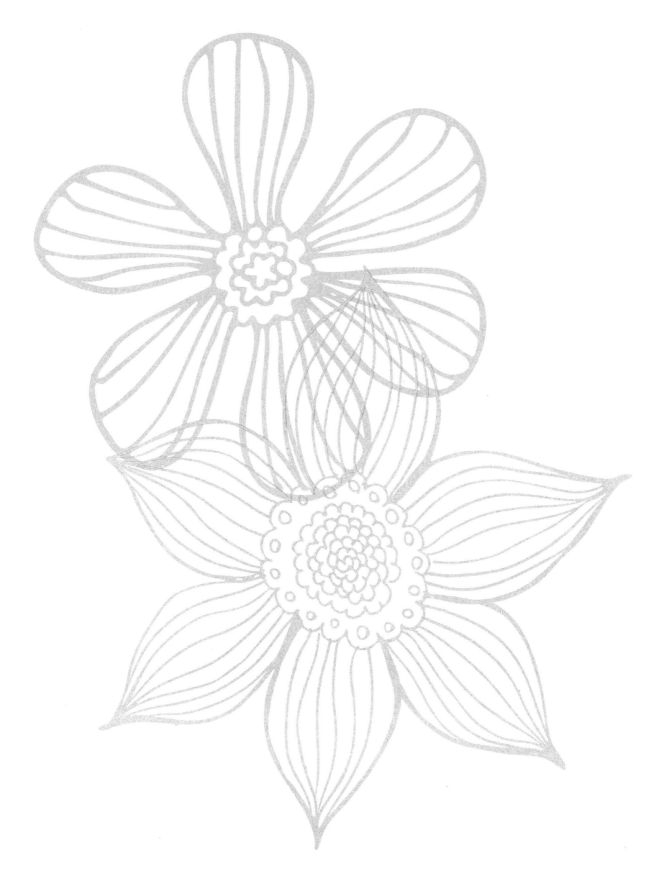

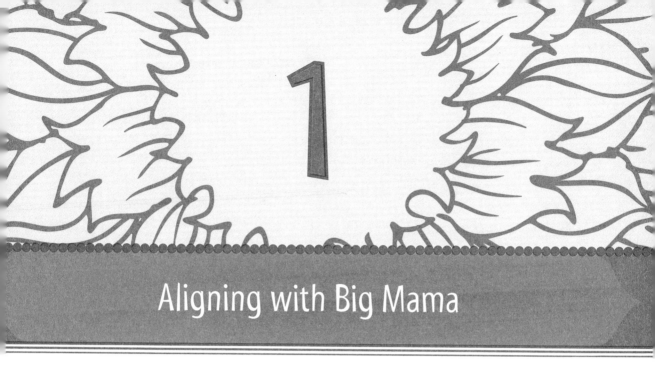

1

Aligning with Big Mama

Ayurveda's view on the science of life is that nothing in this world exists as an isolated entity. We can take things apart as much as we want, but we don't always find clear-cut answers; or as one friend with a PhD in biology put it, "The more I try to take the physical world apart, the more I am left with the same conclusion: Mother Nature is one sneaky lady."

That artful little minx, Mother Nature, has done an excellent job at keeping biologists (and physicists and medical doctors, for that matter) in business. She went ahead and connected everything to everything else. The pint of Häagen-Dazs that you spoon into your mouth this evening could affect how you sleep tonight, what you dream, and how you will feel in the morning. The decision to say no to a social event when you really feel like your body needs to get

10 hours of sleep can provide your immune system with just enough oomph to ward off the gnarly flu that everyone is complaining about. These smaller decisions create both balances and imbalances in the beautiful universe of your body. And wherever there is imbalance in the system, there is disorder and disease. In other words, whatever rocks the boat, rocks the whole sea.

According to Ayurvedic mythology, this everything-is-connected philosophy and practical science emerged out of a deep conversation with God himself (called Brahma in the myth). One day, some wise seers (rishis) were sitting on top of the Himalayas, looking down at the world from their meditative seats. As they watched the human drama below, they started getting frustrated with the state of things. People had no time to live their bliss, to seek their life's purpose, or to truly enjoy the fruits of their hard work. Disease was wreaking havoc on their bodies. Their lifestyles were not in harmony with Nature's rhythms. People couldn't seem to get along, and mental imbalances were a dime a dozen. The worst part of all was that Mother Earth was getting really out of whack. (Sound familiar?)

Because of this chaos, one of the wise seers approached Brahma, asking what could help people. He directly received from God the secrets of Ayurveda. From this one conversation with God, other great teachers were given Ayurvedic knowledge; they were given secrets on how to use massage, oils, herbs, food, lifestyle, and sex (plus many other tools and techniques) to bring humanity back into balance. This book is just one more extension of that first, humbling conversation with God.

Ayurvedic Health

Coming back into balance can mean a number of things for different people, but in general it means that we are healthy, which we all typically define as "a state of well-being free from disease." But this is just one part of health's full picture. Ayurveda describes the state of good health as *svastha*, meaning "established in the soul." In other words, Ayurveda is not just interested in you getting the "perfect body," killer washboard abs, or seeing a certain number when you step on the scale. Its biggest concern is you becoming who the heck you really are. When we are in svastha, we rest in the unchanging center of who we are, which makes us feel good: we feel at home and at ease in our bodies.

Western medicine, while excellent at many things, tends to treat isolated conditions that have already manifested as disease. Ayurveda, on the other hand, focuses on prevention and treating the whole person. Ayurveda embraces the fact that you are unique, with your own idiosyncratic life experiences that have created the unrepeatable woman you are today. A skilled Ayurvedic practitioner would want the lowdown on everything that makes you, well, you.

When I first began to incorporate Ayurveda into my daily life, I was astounded by the strong emphasis self-healing played in the journey toward wellness—and how much self-healing is rooted in knowing oneself. Ayurveda wants us to develop a very close relationship to our own body, our skin, our tongue, our belly, our emotions, as well as the struggles we go through in life, work, sex, and relationships. We are asked to look at these elements of our life as a path toward healing because Ayurveda honors the direct and intertwined relationship between the body's physical health—this flesh and bone thing that we can see and feel—and the mental/emotional body.

Ayurveda asks us to dip into that mental/emotional body by looking at the changing "little me" or egoic self (*asmita*), and identifying with it less. Oh, you know your little me. She is the one that endlessly worries and doubts. She wonders if she will ever have enough money, time, validation, fame, good sex, pairs of shoes. She can't channel her anger and fear into clarity and understanding. She is afraid of stopping long enough to bear witness to her own feelings. She feels guilty for going for her dreams. She envies the good fortune of others. She feels unwanted and unworthy. She is ashamed to ask for what she really wants. She is afraid of being lonely. She ponders, perhaps if only in the silent corners of her heart, whether there really is enough love to go around. She grabs for more when less would do. She believes her life is full of scarcity and negativity, even when abundance is staring her in the face.

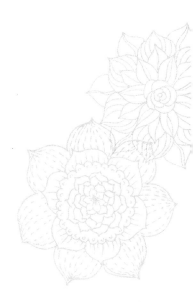

Ayurveda says that unless we move beyond that limited self, we will never taste the golden nectar of real health. You see, Ayurveda views total health as a real and intimate connection to the Big or Higher Self inside us. This Big Self speaks when the little me gets really quiet. You can hear your Big Self as the voice of your intuition telling you to ditch that energy-vampire friend. You can feel her stir when you agree to go out with friends when you really should be resting from last week's flu. She speaks using the language of body sensations, bliss, knowingness, unbounded willpower, and straight-up love.

You may have even been rescued by your Big Self. Remember the last time you felt like you had really hit rock bottom? Then suddenly, as if out of nowhere, there was a voice somewhere saying, "Get up, honey. You've got work to do!" That was your Big Self—the part of you that actually is the Big Mama, All-Knowing, Ass-Kicking, Fear-Busting, Doubt-Dousing, Wise and Spicy, Reverently Orgasmic Cosmic Grandma herself.

The Three Pillars of Health

To be healthy, Ayurveda says that there are three pillars of life that must be honored. The ancient book on Ayurveda, the *Caraka Samhita*, states that there are three supports (pillars) of life. They are food, sleep, and observance of *bramacharya*, the wise use of sexual (or vital) energy. When we are supported by these pillars, the body has good strength, complexion, and growth.[1] In other words, even if you decide not to delve into any of the more mystical undercurrents of Ayurveda, you can still impact your mental and physical well-being by balancing three seemingly simple aspects of your life: food, sleep, and how you use your vital energy.

Sounds great, right? Well, it should be. Food, sleep, and sex are the core ways we nourish ourselves. You may have already had the visceral experience of how a lovingly prepared and well-digested meal, a good night's sleep, and a night of passionate lovemaking—okay, an hour will suffice—with someone you really love can transform your entire outlook on life. This happens because we are being nourished on a number of different levels. You see, Nature delights and rewards us for doing the things that make us feel good, especially when we do them in a healthy way, at the ideal time, and in the proper amount. For example, I love sleeping 8 hours every night. When I'm in balance, I enjoy going to the farmers' market and buying seasonal foods. It makes me feel good, and Nature celebrates those feelings with good health and robust energy. Being Ayurveda-savvy is a practice of getting better at determining which things are going to really make us feel good (deep sleep, healthy food, loving relationships), and letting go of the things that give us a temporary high but deplete us over the long term (double-shot lattes, fast food, and sex without love, for example).

Pillar #1: Food

When diet is wrong, medicine is of no use. When diet is
correct, medicine is of no need.

—**Ayurvedic proverb**

According to Ayurveda, all disease originates in the digestive system. Choosing the right foods for your particular body, as well as the time of day or even the particular season of year, is essential for coming into the feel-good flow. When we eat the wrong foods for our body, eat too much late at night, emotionally eat, or eat winter foods (think butternut squash and stews) in the summer, our belly suffers. In fact, bad digestion could be at the root of much of our social malaise. Millions of people consume fast food and packaged food on a daily basis. Lunch is eaten in cars, in front of computers, or skipped altogether. I know busy moms, corporate go-getters, and even yoga teachers who can't remember if they ate lunch.

Food is the essence of all life. What you put into your body gives you the power to make your life's purpose a reality. In order to be an earth-shaking, present, wise women, we've got to fuel our machine with premium gas.

And Ayurveda does not parse food into calories, vitamins, and minerals. It embraces the holistic energy of different foods and analyzes their qualities (such as hot/cold, light/heavy, dry/wet). Individuals can be analyzed for their qualities as well: Do you tend to run hot or cool? Do you typically feel heavy or light? Is your skin consistently dry or oily? By identifying your own qualities, you can make food choices that are appropriate for your own unique being based on the core Ayurvedic principle of "like increases like." So, for example, if you run hot by nature, avoiding hot, spicy foods might be a good idea. It is also important to know how to prepare and combine foods so that they can be most easily digested. Continually going against what we should eat (both seasonally and constitutionally) leads to imbalance and disease.

Pillar #2: Sleep

Happiness, misery, nourishment, emaciation, strength,
weakness, virility, sterility, knowledge, ignorance,
life and death—all these occur depending on
proper or improper sleep.

—*Caraka Samhita*

If you walk into any pharmacy in America today, you will be over-whelmed by the number of laxatives and sleeping pills on the shelves—laxatives because collective America is chronically constipated, and sleeping pills because we are a nation of acutely sleep-deprived, walking zombies. Combine our toxic overload diet with our sleep deprivation, and there you have it: the state of American health. According to the U.S. Centers for Disease Control and Prevention, when people don't get enough sleep they are more likely to suffer from chronic diseases like hypertension, diabetes, depression, and obesity. The sleep-deprived have also been shown to suffer from higher rates of cancer, reduced quality of life, and lowered productivity at work.[2] With our round-the-clock access to technology, overbooked calendars, and insane work demands, insomnia and other sleep issues are now becoming more the norm than the exception.

Getting our beauty z's can do wonders for how we look and feel, inside and out. Sleep allows the body to detoxify itself from the day, revamping us for the day to come. Sleep is also when we heal the tissues of the physical body. It's the time when we do a major subconscious dump of any undigested emotions and life scenarios. If you currently suffer from insomnia, flip to page 114 for some instant sleep-like-a-baby how-to's.

Pillar #3: Sex

So long as lips shall kiss, and eyes shall see,
so long lives This, and This gives life to Thee.

—**Mallanaga Vātsyāyana, the Kama Sutra**

Ayurvedic practitioners were great believers in the management of sexual energy, valuing what they called bramacharya, or the wise use of this vital sexual energy. When we are using our sexual energy in a harmonious way, our whole life is infused with more enthusiasm around creative projects—whether that be a business, an artistic expression, or a baby. We also have better health in general because Ayurveda sees sexual energy as the most refined aspect of our life energy. The more energy we have, the better we feel.

Ayurveda makes no judgment about sexual expression; there is no right and wrong. It merely encourages us to act wisely in regard to with whom and how we share our sexual energy. Ayurveda understands that men are born with a certain amount of sexual juiciness, and when they run out, it's gone. The good news is that for women, things are a little different. When the body is feeling healthy, it is a good time to enjoy and engage in sexual activity. Orgasms and sexual release do not deplete us as much as they do men. Still, if you are feeling ill or exhausted, taking a temporary sexual sabbatical can be highly beneficial for your body and your energy. Women who are pregnant or breast-feeding may naturally take a pause in sexual activity. This is totally normal and healthy. In the Sexy section of this book, you will learn a lot more about honoring this sacred aspect of your health and womanhood.

More than just sex, this pillar is about vital energy maintenance. How do we use our attention and our body? If we look at one of the meanings of the word *bramacharya*, we gain insight into what the ancients understood. One interpretation of the word is "to walk with God." This is when we try to use our energy in alignment with the Higher Self. An example of this is checking in with our heart (you can think of this as your conscience, intuition, or God) before engaging in decision making. In this way, our choices are more aligned with our highest intentions and the higher good.

Having a healthy womb, and even more importantly, a connection to your physical and energetic sexual centers, is key in boosting this third pillar of health. This book will teach you how to restore the vitality of your sexual energy center and engage in conscious forms

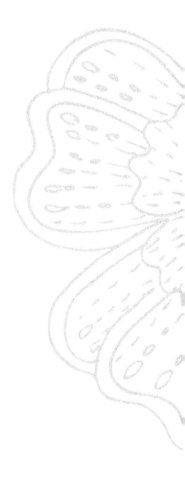

of sacred sexuality. When a woman feels tuned in to her sacred sexual essence, a new aliveness begins to pulse within her. Her health improves. Her eyes glimmer. And all of Creation is at her disposal.

Tattoo This on Your Fridge

When we are balanced, our senses actually feed our good choices, and we become more tuned toward balance. When we are out of balance, they send us toward the people, places, foods, and forms of entertainment that bring us into deeper states of imbalance. Personally, I know I'm in balance when I start craving steamed broccoli, early nights with a good book, and positive social connection with my family.

The first way we get out of balance is through upset in the digestive system (whether we notice it or not). Weak digestion creates something called *ama*. We can approximate its translation in English as "toxins." When you don't digest things well, they build up in the system and turn rotten. Think of ama as a slimy, beige-colored toxic sludge that smothers the movement of energy in your digestive tract. In the body, this manifests as bloating, weight gain, acne, fatigue, constipation, and many other unsavory symptoms. (Chapter 6 will cover this in detail.)

We can experience mental/emotional ama as well. This ama is the accumulation of undigested life experiences that blocks the channels of our perception; it is the storehouse of our negativity stories. You can measure how full your storehouse is by looking at how much you blame others for your current life circumstances or how often you get offended by people, politics, or the weather conditions; when you find these things happening more often and more easily, you have a buildup of ama. Ama is like sludgy mind-mucus dripping down from your brain and putting out the fire of sweetness in your heart.

Sometimes imbalances occur as a natural result of the environment we live in. Ama can accumulate, for example, if we live in polluted air or drink polluted water. Sometimes we experience disease as a natural process of aging and decay. If you leave a metal chair outside for a few years, the environment and time will age it. Our bodies are the same. Happily, Ayurveda teaches us how to slow down the natural pull of decay so that we can stay vital and gleaming longer. The body is limited. Over time, the body begins to decay due to the sheer force of death itself.

The good news is that Ayurveda gives us the basics of how to fool the Grim Reaper for as long as possible while simultaneously delighting in the physical realm. Ayurveda understands the important role that the mind plays in how the body experiences time. The more we speed down the road, jacked up on coffee while frantically texting our

Founder of Jivamukti Yoga, Sharon Gannon's First Experience of Ayurveda

My first experience with Ayurvedic healing happened in the early nineties. I was in a small town in South India. The air was stifling. It was the afternoon, and I was sitting on a rusty metal bench in a tiny, dirt-floor room with four other people all waiting to see the doctor. I had come with a friend of mine to offer support. She hadn't been feeling well for the past week or so. She said that her body ached all over; she had lost interest in food and found it difficult to get out of bed in the morning. She felt not only physically tired, but also emotionally depressed, with a recurring feeling of "what's the use?" hanging over her like a dark cloud. Finally, the doctor called us into his office. He asked her what was wrong, and my friend told him how she had been feeling. He then asked her a matter-of-fact question: "So, madam, do you want to feel better?"

To which she replied, "Yes."

"Okay then get up. Spread your feet apart, stand up straight, release your arms by your sides," he commanded in a heavy Indian accent, and although somewhat startled by his tone of voice, she obeyed. "Now start the shaking of your body, lift your right foot off the floor, and shake it, then your left, now each hand and arm, shake your head, let your jaw relax, move around—move, move—get down on the floor and roll around—move, come on, don't stop— shake all over."

He had her movin' and shakin' for a good five minutes without a stop, while I just sat in a corner and watched. Then he said, "Okay, you will feel better now, please give me twenty rupees." We paid and walked out of the Ayurvedic clinic—both of us laughing uncontrollably. My friend was cured of her malaise by moving her body. You could say she shook her sickness off."

(For Sharon Gannon's full contribution to *Healthy Happy Sexy*, check out www.healthyhappysexylife.com.)

significant others because we forgot to pick up one of the kids, the more our aging clock speeds up. The more present and calm we are, the more that clock chills out. Stress ages us, so if you want to look younger, you would do well to throw out the plethora of antiaging creams you spent last month's salary on, and start hanging out in the present moment.

There is a deep interconnection in our moment-to-moment choices and our wellness. It may sound too easy, but by simply slowing down, we can start to pay attention to our own three pillars of health—food, sleep, and sex. When we slow down and eat wholesome foods, we sleep better. When we sleep better, we don't crave as many sugary, high-carb snacks for energy. And when we feel healthy and well-rested, our sexual energy can flow in the best of ways. Over and over, I have found in myself, and my clients and students, that a complicated life calls for very simple remedies and solutions. Oftentimes, simply paying attention to the three pillars of health is enough to correct many health challenges. Our body's wisdom takes over and our vitality, happiness, and sexiness just flow naturally.

• • Essential Ideas • •

- Ayurveda says that when we are balanced in the three pillars of health, we will make more balanced choices. When we are out of balance, we seek more imbalance.
- There are three Ayurvedic pillars of health: food, sleep, and sex.
- Bramacharya is the intelligent use of our sexual, vital, energy.
- When we are in balance, we avoid ama, the buildup of toxins, both physical and emotional.

Putting Ayurveda to Work

Balancing your three pillars may first require some letting go of the "busy" factor in your life. Get out your journal and answer the following: Where in your life can you simplify? What commitments are vital and which can be dropped? Where are you saying yes, when you really want to say no? How are you going to use your creative potential and sexual vitality this week in new and inspiring ways? Roll out a canvas to paint on. Start a garden. Take a pleasurable bath. If you are in a relationship, you can also work with your partner on deepening intimacy. Anyone can boost this creative force and tune to the sensuality and aliveness of existence.

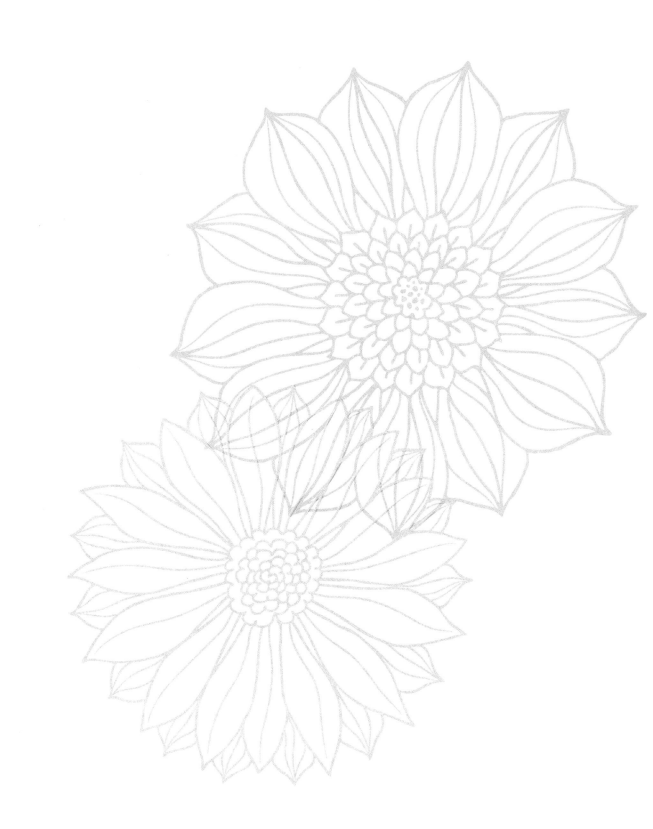

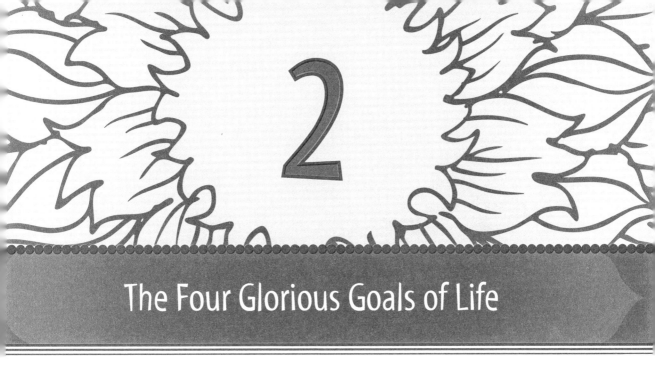

The Four Glorious Goals of Life

There is a strong connection between staying healthy in the three pillars mentioned in chapter 1 and our soul's ability to thrive and be happy. When our digestion is good, our sleep is deep and our emotions and sexuality are being channeled properly. We have more energy to engage in our passions and pursuits in life—in Ayurveda, our foremost pursuits are known as the four goals of life.

According to the Vedas (the spiritual root texts of Ayurveda), your soul has four goals or desires, which the texts call the *purusharthas*, "that which is for the purpose of the soul." The Ayurvedic tradition takes these four core human motivations and gives us permission to enjoy and pursue them, while not becoming overly attached to any of them. In this way, we can enjoy pleasure, seek success and purpose, strive for material gain, and seek out the practices and mentors that will teach us how to live a more integrated, enlightened, soulful life. By no means will my general overview do justice to the complex tapestry of what these four motivators are or how we can succeed in their fulfillment, but I do hope to give a brief summary, as they are paramount in our sense of total health and happiness. (For more on these glorious goals and how to manifest them in your life, check out the book *The Four Desires* by Rod Stryker.)

Life Goal #1: Luscious, Everyday Pleasure

The first goal of life is *kama*, meaning pleasure or enjoyment. (Surely you've heard of the Kama Sutra! A sutra is a teaching, making the Kama Sutra the "pleasure teachings.") If we are to live life fully, we need life to feel good. There is nothing like the sensory stimulation we get from smelling a baby's skin, stroking a kitten's silky fur, seeing a peony in full bloom, or running a hand over a man's deltoid muscle. What brings you deep sensory satisfaction?

Start Now: The Pleasure Principle Meditation

Start by closing your eyes. Slowly let your breath become smooth and even. Bring your attention to the sensations in your belly. Keep your awareness anchored at your navel and feel the way the inhale expands your belly away from your spine. Feel the way your exhale draws your belly back toward your spine. When you are deeply relaxed, bring your attention to each of your five sensory organs: sight, smell, hearing, taste, and touch. Contemplate your sensual capacity as a gift from the Divine. Spend some time really feeling your skin and its ability to perceive sensations. Notice the subtle smells, sounds, and even the taste inside your mouth. Open your eyes and just spend a minute noticing the colors, the light, and the more subtle aspects of your sight. The Divine wants you to experience the beauty of this world and the miracles of creation through these gateways. When you feel the pleasure inherent in the five senses, you have touched your first longing, kama.

The great news is that Nature has set it up so that many of the things that feel good to us are also physiologically and emotionally good for us. Science shows that touch (whether a massage therapist's or a lover's) increases the hormones in our body that keep our immune system functioning.[1] It's a downright miracle that just the smell of onions simmering in olive oil causes our body to release the very digestive enzymes that it will use to process the food when we eat it. That's Divine Intelligence and Mama Nature's way of saying, "Relish this moment!"

The problem with all this wonderful kama comes when we overindulge. Remember in *Charlie and the Chocolate Factory* when Augustus Gloop ends up as a piece of fudge after falling into the river of chocolate? Without proper guidance, the out-of-balance, overindulging aspect of our senses can ignore our internal attempts at regulation. If we leave our senses in the driving seat, we run the risk of overdoing it—whether it be booze, chocolate, shopping, sex, TV, or exercise.

The secret to true fulfillment in the realm of pleasure is self-awareness, moderation, and nonattachment. Nonattachment has not always been an easy thing for me to practice. When I enjoy something, I sometimes wanna hold on. Talking to the Divine has helped me build a form of surrender. Whenever I feel myself clinging to pleasures, I will stop and say something like, "Oh, Divine Mama, let me trust in your infinite abundant sources. May I know that this pleasure may rise and fall, but that you are continually dropping your grace into my life." When we cling, it is as though we don't believe in all that the Universe offers; it is as if we are saying that we don't have faith that pleasure (or whatever it is we want to cling to) is abundant and always waiting for us. It helps me to simply pay attention. I know that I don't need to cling because when I'm paying attention, I see that the beauty is always being offered to me.

Another way to practice nonattachment is to be deeply aware of the present moment while enjoying pleasure. Think of it as simultaneously relishing and releasing.

Life Goal #2: The Means for Prospering

The second goal of life is *artha*, or the ways and means of prosperous living. Artha is related to the tools that help us move forward in life. A place to live, enough money to pay the bills, good health, proper clothing, and even your iPhone are all examples of tools that help you move through life with more ease.

Just as we want pleasure, we also love the feeling of abundance and good health. It feels good to rest easy, knowing that our basic needs are met. It's hard to think about the meaning of life when we are pawning our jewelry or arguing with credit card company minions. Ayurveda encourages us not only to pursue financial abundance, but it also states that without a certain sense of ease around finances, our advancement toward knowing who we are is hindered. Why? Because if we are worried about finances, our mind becomes easily disturbed, fearful, and distracted. A similar thing happens with our health. If we are sick, it's hard to meditate, help our kids with their homework, or launch our dream business.

Imbalance in artha occurs when we become greedy or too focused on materialism. When we have 13 shades of lip-plumping lipstick and yet feel positive we really need one more, we may have an accumulation problem. I will never forget walking into my neighbor's house. She had amassed 157 stuffed animals. Shoes (still in their boxes) were stacked from floor to ceiling, wall-to-wall. She had a guest room full of purses (piled on a virtually invisible bed, price tags still attached to many of them). The primary motivating force in her life had become acquiring things. She had slowly built up a safety bubble composed of teddy bears, high heels, and handbags. I think that if we are honest, many of us have a little bit of the crazy-teddy-bear lady inside us. Ayurveda teaches us how to embrace our love for stuffed animals without smothering ourselves with them.

Artha can also be imbalanced when we mistakenly think that we need nothing. I know a few spiritual people who feel wrong or guilty for wanting nice things, like a warm home, soft clothing, or a chocolate bar (even if it's organic, fair-trade). This is the opposite end of the artha spectrum, and it is just as harmful for our total wellness. The lesson? It's okay to need things—in moderation and for the purpose of the higher good.

Life Goal #3:
Roll Out of Bed with a Purpose

The third goal of life is *dharma*, or our essential life purpose. In the craziness of daily life, many of us forget what a mind-blowing opportunity it is to be in a human body (as opposed to being born a honey badger). Ayurveda says that every human being comes into this life with a specific dharma, and until we are living that dharma, we will not be happy. My teacher, Rod Stryker, says there is a you-shaped hole in the Universe just waiting to be filled. Until you figure out how to embody your full expression and purpose, you will feel out of sync with what your Higher Self longs to become.

Dharmic pursuits do not necessarily have to fulfill any holier-than-thou requirements, however. Dharma has nothing to do with what we could call "a job," but is more likened to the unique thing you bring to the table in any of life's circumstances (be it a job, a relationship or a project). What is more, people working in jobs that may not have cachet in society can be quite important on the cosmic scene. For example, have you ever met someone with what our society may consider a lowly or bad job, yet she seems to be totally in love with it? Or she uses it to make your day better? That is the embodiment of someone living her dharma.

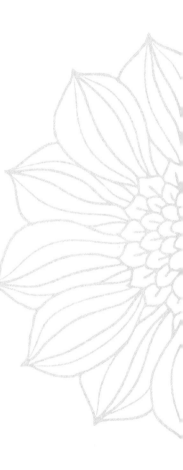

I remember going into a bathroom at the airport one day. Inside stood a woman whose sole job it was to make sure there was sufficient toilet paper, the sinks were clean, and the towel machines were working. As soon as I walked in, I was blasted with, "Hi, honey, how are you? You look beautiful today!"

I imagined the other trip-weary women inside those stalls pulling up their pantyhose to the music of her blessings.

"Have a blessed day, honey!" she reminded me as I left.

And you know what? She made it a much better day. In fact, her generous compassion has stayed inside of me to this day. Now you are reading about her. She is traveling out into the world over space and time! There she stood in a public restroom all day long, saying the same thing over and over. It could have been the standard, "Hello, how are you?" But instead, this woman embodied delight. She used her work as a way to connect, uplift, and remind us that even within the smelly confines of an airport bathroom we have an opportunity to share our essential goodness.

In order to align with our essential life purpose, we need enough balance to actually hear the inner voice of our intuition. Most people who are fully working in their passion will tell you that they had no choice; their job chose them. They say they feel a kinetic flow of energy when they are working in the realm of what they love. Researchers such as Mihaly Csikszentmihalyi are now confirming the existence of a creative psychological flow space that people enter when they are working in their dharma. Time seems to slow, even stop. Energy levels are high, and there is a feeling of aliveness and presence that gives us even more motivation for the work at hand. Feeling this flow space is a good indication that we are aligned with our dharma and in what Csikszentmihalyi calls the optimal experience in his book *Flow*.

A technique for aligning with your personal life purpose is to ask yourself, *If I had limitless finances and time, what would I be doing right now?* If you are living your dharma, you will answer, *Exactly what I am doing.* If not, it may be time to reassess your life purpose. Ayurvedic lifestyle tools help us align with our dharma by bringing the body and mind into balance. Meditation is key, as it allows us to get quiet enough to move beyond the fears and doubts that keep us from moving toward what is most right for us—and for the world.

Start Now: What's in the Way of Discovering Your Dharma?

- Get 2 pieces of paper and a pen.
- Start by contemplating and then completing this sentence: "If I had unlimited time and finances, I would _____." (For example, "I would be traveling the world taking photos of rare exotic birds.")
- Write down your answer, then take a moment to envision yourself doing exactly what you wrote down.
- Now write your answer, using the present tense, over and over for 5 minutes. ("I travel the world taking photos of rare exotic birds.") Notice what resistance comes up as you continue, and write these thoughts down on another sheet of paper as they arise ("I would never have the money to be able to do this." "My mother would think this was a total waste of time." "I will never get health insurance if I leave my current job.")

Ayurvedic teachings say that there are entities of negativity sitting inside our mind-field, literally pulling us away from the things we love. Your job is to loosen the hold these negative statements have on you and release your belief in them. Take a few moments now to write some phrases that counteract the negativity. (To continue our example, the statement "No one cares about my silly photographs of birds" could be counteracted with "My passion for endangered birds translates into my work and is valued financially and artistically.")

Life Goal #4: Give Me Liberty

The fourth goal of life is *moksha*, or freedom. Ultimately, behind all of our actions lies the drive to move beyond the recurring cycles of pain/pleasure and birth/death, and to feel the happiness of not being subject to these polarities. Moksha is waking up in the morning and feeling fearless. Moksha is the sense that there is nothing out there that will bring us ultimate happiness—it's all inside ourselves. Moksha is truly needing nothing and no one to be whole and complete.

The farther we advance on the path of knowing who we are, the more this goal becomes clear and the more we can align our life choices with things that will support our own true freedom. If we become too attached to the idea of freedom, we run the danger of becoming a holier-than-thou, spiritual egoist. I have seen students and friends attempt freedom through the path of what psycho-spiritual experts call "spiritual bypassing," basically attempting to run away from the "bad" world by checking out into some flaky spiritual zone where we don't deal with our issues. The teachings state that this is impossible. We can't run away from pain or pleasure, birth or death, or even our own internal struggles (karmas). What we can do is learn how to become a loving witness to all of life's duality.

Real moksha is about tapping in. It's about seeing the bigger picture, what life looks like beyond our own motivations. You can measure your success in the realm of moksha by how fearlessly and joyfully you live your life in this current, imperfect world, as well as how well you surrender your negative feelings when you don't get what you want. It's also about seeing things as they really are and moving beyond the material world. But the stuff that flashes on billboards, the phone calls, the dinner dates, the news, and the warm touch of a loved one are all very real to us, so the more we work toward knowing who we are, the more we can delight in the existence of this illusory, temporary world of the senses, while at the same time experiencing the Divine delight behind it all. In this sense, we become free because we are fully and delightfully engaged with the temporal beauty of life as it is unfolding.

Ayurveda is compassionate with our hearts. Why? Because these four goals act as sweet reminders that the heart has deep, and perhaps even hidden, desires. Use these four desires as the cornerstone upon which your health and well-being can rest. When we make these desires a foundation point, we begin to live a more complete and balanced life. Our soul begins to thrive at many different levels of existence— physical, sensual, intellectual, and spiritual. Perhaps most importantly, this teaching forms the backbone for feeling truly joyful and deeply fulfilled. And when you thrive and feel happy, you can be sure that the whole world feels the contribution of your soul, and in turn becomes a better place to live. There is nothing more beautiful and more sexy than a woman who is deeply fulfilled.

• • Essential Ideas • •

- There are four main human goals or desires: kama (pleasure), artha (prosperity), dharma (purpose), and moksha (freedom).
- When we feel fulfilled in all the goals, we are happy. When any of the four is lacking, we feel that lack.
- When we are thriving in the world and spiritually fulfilled, we make the world a better place to live.

Putting Ayurveda to Work

Sit quietly somewhere. Get out your journal and answer the following questions: how are you currently thriving in each of these four life pursuits? Which of these desires does your heart crave the most? Once you have your answer, brainstorm on some concrete ways that you can fulfill that desire. Put this statement in the present tense. Here are some examples of daily, weekly, or monthly commitments to fulfilling your longings:

- Every day, I dance to my favorite music for 15 minutes because it brings me great pleasure.
- Rob and I have date night once a week, just the two of us. Once every 3 months we go away for the weekend.
- I am volunteering at the homeless shelter once a month.
- I work on my screenplay for 30 minutes every day.
- I have $20,000 in my savings account by saving $500 monthly.

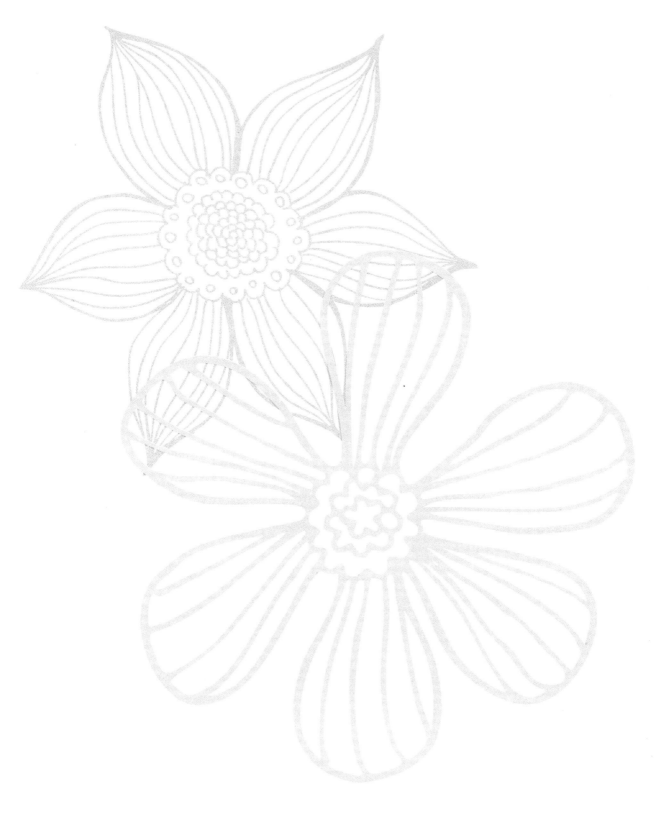

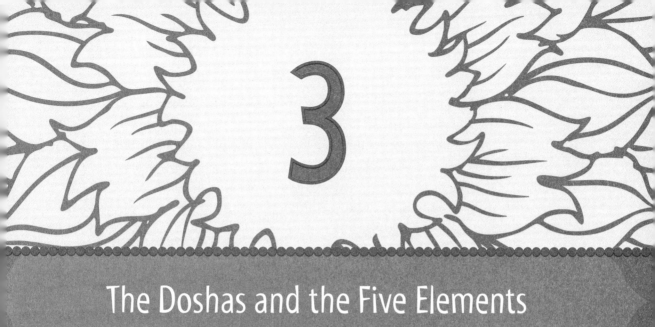

3

The Doshas and the Five Elements

The more balanced we are in the essential pillars of health (food, sleep, and sex), the more we can thrive in the realms of our four essential goals: pleasure, prosperity, purpose, and freedom. Now we can go even deeper into the Ayurvedic view of health, happiness, and sexual vitality. In order to experience an even stronger connection to our highest wellness, we have to get down into the elemental nature of who we are. Ayurveda teaches that the whole world, from the tallest mountain to the tiniest atom in the body, is composed of five essential elements, all of which were born of a deep, cosmic love affair. That means that, in essence, the outer world is completely reflected within the individual.

This chapter is all about helping you understand how this elemental love affair is expressed in your individual body and mind.

An Ode to the Elements

Ether, Air, Fire, Water, and Earth—these elemental love babies of the Universe are constantly at play in both the physical and nonphysical realms. Together they create the world we experience with our senses. The five elements are also the forces behind all the physical processes in our own bodies. It may be hard at first to imagine these elements in your own body, but you can start by thinking of them as metaphors for the processes inside you. With time and practice, you will become familiar with them and feel them in your body and mind.

By understanding the nature of the five elements, we see how they interact with one another to create both balance and imbalance. Thinking of yourself in terms of these elements will give you a foundation for discovering your mind-body type. Through the five elements, we relate to ourselves as natural and unique expressions of nature. By understanding nature's play inside us as a unique combination of all five of these elements, we can achieve greater balance. Typically, we are strongly composed of 1–2 of these elements, with side helpings of the rest. When you read about each of them, look for clues as to which elements you tend to embody.

Ether

Ether is the space that exists between things. It is defined as the absence of the other four elements. It is the fabric upon which the Divine story is written. Ether is so subtle that we cannot perceive it with our five senses but we know when it is there, and we seriously miss it when it is absent. On a physical level, Ether is represented by the cavities or empty spaces that exist in the body, such as the space in the lungs or the cavity of the stomach. We feel mentally spacious when we can see an array of possibilities for ourselves; we are spacious when we are not bogged down by the minutia of daily tasks and can see the bigger picture.

The lesson of Ether: sacred space. Make space for silence. Own an entire space in your home (even if it's a cleared-out closet that you sneak into once a day). Clear your calendar one day a week, or at least a few days each month. Let the spaciousness in your calendar lead you to spontaneous action and creation. Meditate to clear the space of your mind and emotions. Take a trip alone to get some time (which is also space) away from family duties and responsibilities.

Air

Air is not only the principle of movement and change; it is also that which sets all events into motion. If you are having trouble getting a project off the ground, you may need to cultivate a little more Air in your life. And don't be fooled by the lightness of Air. If you have ever been in a hurricane or a tornado, you know that air can be one of the most powerful forces on the planet. In the body, Air governs the movement of the nerve impulses, the breath, and the movement of our limbs. In the mind, Air moves thought. Too much Air can leave us feeling hyper-mobile. You may have experienced this as a longing to nest in your home after too much travel.

The lesson of Air: embrace change. Celebrate that which you did not plan. Take inventory of how much enthusiasm you feel toward your life. Are you living in a way that challenges you to become a bigger version of yourself? If not, start to make a list of all your unfulfilled longings. What new wind inside you is longing to take flight?

Fire

We need Fire to transform our lives. Without Fire, our life may feel stagnant. We have all felt the heaviness and inertia of a lack of motivation. Too much Fire, on the other hand, can leave us feeling burned out or raw from the sheer transformational force of life. Perhaps witnessing the death of a loved one has left you feeling forever altered and worn out by the shock. When Fire is too strong, we can come back to both Ether (spaciousness) to reduce Fire's intensity, as well as Water (to cool the flames).

The lesson of Fire: let life slowly burn you. When life becomes challenging, we know we are in the Fire. Life burns us to humble us, and humility is the salve that heals the wounds on an aching ego. Fire brings wisdom by melting away everything that we are not. The quieter we become, the more we can rest in the wise and most compassionate One, the infinitely beautiful One, the One that is our own spirit. When life is challenging, sit with the Fire and let the wisdom emerge. When emotions arise, feel them deeply.

Water

We need Water to lubricate our lives with sweetness. Without Water, our life may feel like it lacks pleasure and sensuality. Too much Water, on the other hand, can leave us feeling unambitious and lazy. We can also be dominated by Water's unconscious sensuality, allowing attachments to rule our otherwise logical and intuitive knowingness.

The lesson of Water: go with the flow. Practice surfing the waves of life with grace and compassion. Emotions are very watery creatures. They rise and fall, taking up the container of the body, washing us clean from a misguided perspective or an old holding pattern. In the ebb and flow of events and emotions, know that you are completely loved and protected. To fully receive the gifts of Water, let everything wash over you like an ocean wave.

Earth

Earth is the principle of stability and the solidity of matter. It is the quality that makes up the firmness of wood, metal, a blade of grass, or your calf muscles. In the body, Earth represents physical structure. In the mind, Earth represents mental and emotional stability. Stability does not mean you aren't rattled or, at times, broken. It means that despite the chaos of life, there is a foundational part of you that knows you will be fine.

The lesson of Earth: I am worthy. Earth tells us that we are worthy of being here, with the full weight of our presence. It teaches us to stand firm and be confident about who we are. When your confidence wanes, engage in activities that build Earth. Surround yourself with a loving community, lift weights, grind spices, dance on the earth with your feet, plant a garden, dig a hole.

Ayurvedic Doshas

The elements are inanimate on their own. They have to mix! And when they mix, they become life forces that take on different forms and movement. These forces are called the *tri-doshas*, and they are key in learning how to practically address your health and well-being in everyday life.

A *dosha* can be defined as particular patterns of energy that create your unique physical, emotional, and mental being. They are patterns of intelligence that govern your body, emotions, and mind. Dosha literally translates as "fault" (as in fault line) or "forces that easily go out of balance." These doshas are the forces that cause things to happen inside and through us, minute by minute. And on the macro level, they are the natural forces of Mother Nature that keep our world in constant movement, transformation, and (temporary) stability. These energies are so potent, so powerful (think nuclear reactor) that our inner Divine Mama spends a large amount of time trying to balance them out. And while we love to fault the doshas for easily going out of balance, it is because of these imbalances that life exists at all!

There are three primary doshas at work in all of us: *vata*, *pitta*, and *kapha*. Vata is the force that moves things in you. It is kinetic energy, related to movement, breath, and elimination. Pitta is the force that digests things in you. It is metabolic energy, related to assimilation and transformation. Kapha is the force that holds things together in you. It is potential energy, related to stability and lubrication.

Discovering Your Dosha Type

Have you ever noticed how your friends are all delightfully different? For example, my friend Kate is a stone-cold fox, like a hipster Audrey Hepburn. She seems cool, calm, and collected even after a week at Burning Man. She eats mangos wrapped in smoked salmon and never has a digestive complaint. Meanwhile, I miss a few hours of precious sleep or eat one dinner past eight o'clock, and I feel like a walking zombie with a bloated tummy. Is life unfair? Well, yes and no. You see, each of us is predisposed to certain imbalances due to our elemental makeup. The good news is that our elemental makeup also allows us to embody different and beautiful capacities.

Each of us is born with our own individual—and perfect—combination of all three, with usually one dominant dosha. Some mystics believe that our original dosha balance was given to us as a means for fulfilling our particular purpose in the world. Sometimes through our hectic lives and less-than-ideal food choices, that original balance is lost. Our goal is to reestablish the balance we had at birth. Typically, you will have one dosha that is strongest, however, some people have proportionate amounts of two (bi-doshic), and other very rare people have all three in proportion (tri-doshic).

As we go through the doshas, put a little check beside all the qualities you identify with, no matter which dosha it belongs to. Then count up your checks to see how much of each of the doshas you embody to identify your dominant one. You might want to ask a close friend or family member to look over your checklist. For example, you might think you don't need to check the box that reads "Frequently gets irritable," but your best friend may think otherwise! Keep it real, mama—this is for your own good!

Vata Dosha

The first dosha is vata, or "that which moves things." Vata is the part of us associated with the elements of Air and Ether. She is a beautiful, moving mess. She is the wind of change in the body. Like a wild artist with unstoppable creativity, she has the qualities of lightness, movement, change, roughness, quickness, and dryness. Physically, vata is the force behind the nervous system, respiration, and elimination. You may have experienced imbalanced vata energy if you have had dry skin, constipation, premature wrinkles, anxiety, fear or a general feeling of being spaced out.

At the level of the mind and spirit, when we use our powerful vata for good, we embody the pure expression of enthusiasm for life. In fact, the word enthusiasm comes from the Greek root *theos*, meaning "God," and *en*, meaning "within." Therefore, the beauty of a person with a dominant vata nature lies in their ability to express a genuine enthusiasm for the God within. When in balance, vata people make excellent healers, inspired writers and artists, and enthusiastic speakers.

Fill this out for your long-term tendencies, not necessarily how you feel today. Think of how you have felt/lived/been over your entire life, not just this week.

You may have more vata if:

- You have a slimmer frame body with a fine bone structure and unpronounced muscles.
- You tend to have a hard time putting on weight.
- You have drier skin.
- You tend toward constipation or gas or both when your digestion is off. ✓
- You have premature wrinkles.
- You have been called spacy or even an airhead. ✓
- You have a wonderfully creative mind and can change your mind easily. ✓
- Your speech is fast, with an exuberant or nervous tone, and you can be a drama queen when you talk. ✓
- You are capable of original thought, and you are an artist, musician, or inventor. ✓
- You have thinner and finer hair, small eyes, and more brittle nails.
- Your voice has been called "airy" and may have a thinner, higher tonality.
- Your appetite varies and your eyes are often bigger than your belly.
- You are a super-quick learner, but if you are out of balance it can go in one ear and out the other unless you really focus. ✓
- You like airy foods like toast, chips, and crackers. ✓
- You have the tendency to multitask.
- When you're out of balance, you tend toward anxiety and nervousness, or fear and depression. ✓
- You have been called a worrywart. ✓
- You have an urge toward deep spiritual practice, esotericism and/or asceticism. ✓
- You are drawn to dabble in mind-altering drugs.
- You have deep intuition or even some psychic abilities. ✓
- Your resting pulse ranges from 80 to 100 beats per minute.

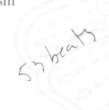

- Your sleep is light and when you are out of balance, you are prone to early-morning insomnia. ✓
- You bite your nails.
- You feel too cold more often than too hot. ✓
- You have an irregular menstrual cycle or scanty menstruation.
- You spend money as fast as it comes in.
- You have quick, active, and/or fearful dreams.

Pitta Dosha

The second dosha is pitta, or "that which digests things." I see pitta as a glowingly hot arrow. She is the heat of transformation. She is the energy of Fire and a little Water. You may have experienced pitta's imbalanced side when you have had fever, loose stools, skin rash or acne, or the heated emotions of anger and frustration.

Pitta has the qualities of sharpness, oiliness, lightness, and instability. In the physical body, pitta is behind our digestion and metabolism. It is force of heat in the body that keeps us at a sultry 98.6°F. On the plane of the mind and spirit, pitta carries the gift of discernment that can cut through the smokescreen, allowing you to see a situation clearly.

You know your mental pitta is weak, for example, if you continually repeat the same life errors over and over again (I think of dating). The mental aspect of pitta is weak if we keep meeting the same emotionally unavailable men over and over again. You will know your mental fire is getting stronger when you can quickly sift the wheat from the chaff—and do so with grace and kindness. This applies not only to discernments about lovers, but also to the decisions we make about friendship, jobs, and even the types of food we buy. When we use our pitta fire for good, we have the ability to see the white-hot truth about ourselves and others. When it is out of balance, we become overly critical and compulsive—like those people who insist on rearranging others' emotional spice cabinets or micromanaging a grown child's life path.

You may have more pitta if:

- You have a naturally muscular/toned body, with a medium bone structure. ✓
- You have a more angular face, with deep set, moderately sized eyes. ✓
- You have slightly oily skin, with a rosy or ruddy complexion. ✓
- Your skin is sensitive, possibly prone to rashes or acne.
- You tend toward looser stools when your digestion is off.
- Your hair started turning gray early.
- You have been called intense.
- You have a wonderfully sharp, focused mind and often feel that you know the best way to do things. ✓
- You have leadership qualities and it's difficult for you to be a follower when in a group setting. ✓
- You have finer hair that is light in color.
- Your appetite is strong. You have been known to get "hangry" (hungry + angry).
- You are often thirsty. ✓
- When you skip a meal or are hungry, your friends know to watch out as you may become angry or irritated. ✓
- When you are out of balance, you crave spicy foods.
- When you are mentally or emotionally out of balance, you tend toward intensity, anger or irritation. You can also be highly critical of others and yourself. ✓
- Your menstrual cycle is regular, with a medium to moderate flow.
- You feel too hot more often than too cold.
- Your speech is moderately paced, your tone is sharp or intense, and your words can be combative or judgmental when you are out of balance.
- Your resting pulse ranges from 70 to 80 beats per minute.
- You have very colorful dreams, sometimes with fiery elements like war or violence.
- You love spending money on luxuries.

Kapha Dosha

The third dosha is kapha, or "that which holds things together." Luscious and well-lubricated, kapha is the ancient dependability of a mountain, the stable womb of a mama's belly, or the absolute trust of a family dinner ritual. I see her as the soft, big-breasted mother archetype, sturdy down to the bone, consistent as the rising sun. Kapha is the combined elements of Earth and Water. It is the meat, fat, liquid, and bones of the body, the parts that keep us strong and well oiled. Kapha is also the force behind the lymphatic system and the mucous membranes. It is related to the qualities of stability, heaviness, wetness, and coolness.

On a subtler front, kapha is related to holding on. When it is out of balance, that holding on can turn into gripping or a codependent attachment. Has anyone ever accused you of "smothering" them with your love? This may be an indication of some kapha in your constitution. Kaphas are also the ones who still have every love letter that their middle school boyfriend ever wrote them, and may keep a zoo-full of stuffed animals on their beds. Although all three doshas can experience weight gain, kapha types have the hardest time losing excess weight (and the easiest time gaining it).

You may have more kapha if:

- You have a thicker build and a rounder face.
- You sometimes say, "If I just look at food, I gain weight."
- You have rounder body features in general.
- Your cheeks are plump and your nose is fleshy.
- Your eyes are large and round. You have been told that they are unbelievably beautiful.
- You have been told that you have great skin. People have asked to touch it, as it is wonderfully soft. Your skin can be moist and, when out of balance, have cystic acne.
- You have strong, healthy gums and teeth.
- Your hair is thick, curly, wavy, and/or has a polished look.
- Your joints are large and well lubricated. They don't ache or crunch or squeak. They are not prone to inflammation.

- You are rarely super thirsty.
- Your appetite is predictable, but not necessarily big.
- You tend toward slower digestion and may feel heavy after eating. ✓
- Your stools tend to be large and bulky, possibly even with mucus.
- You sweat a lot, but it smells sweet.
- You have been called earthy or grounded. Your friends know that they can always count on you.
- You are a total love bug, but you can get possessive or overly sentimental when out of balance. ✓
- You are generally calm and consistent. ✓
- When out of balance, you may be a hoarder.
- Your body temperature tends to be cool, but not cold.
- Your period is regular with an average to heavy flow. ✓
- You sleep heavily when in balance. You love sleeping late and it can be hard to get out of bed in the morning.
- Your speech moves at a slow pace, your tone is soft, and your words are usually sweet.
- Your resting pulse ranges from 60 to 70 beats per minute. Closest
- Your dreams are romantic. You dream of sex, snow, and watery places like cool mountain lakes.
- You have good finances and know how to save money.

Your Constitution

When you were born, you were a perfect blend of the specific combination of the five elements (Ether, Air, Fire, Water, and Earth) that make up your unique dosha. Just as every person on this planet has a unique set of fingerprints, your elemental nature is a wild and wonderful "fingerprint" that is unique to you. The combination of the elements you were born with is called your *prakruti* [PRA-KROO-TEE], a term that means "nature" or "first creation." This means that if you were born a big-boned brunette with bright green eyes and a tendency to have a short fuse, there is little likelihood that you will become a thin-framed, brown-eyed blond with the natural patience of an oak tree. (Okay, you could bleach your hair, get colored contacts, and practice a lot of meditation, but those gorgeous big bones are yours for life.)

As we grow and move through life, some of our inborn traits may remain consistent, but with the passing of the years, most of us move further out of balance. This happens for a number of reasons. Here are a few:

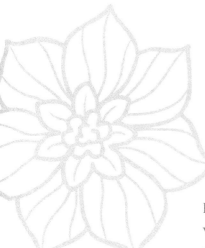

- Being in a soul-sucking job
- Moving so quickly in life that our emotions don't get channeled and expressed appropriately
- Feeling isolated/alone
- Not eating home-cooked, nourishing food
- Being in toxic relationships
- Being a mother without real support
- Feeling that you aren't living your true purpose, or not expressing an art or talent that needs to be expressed

So What Dosha Am I?

First of all, you have an original dosha (prakruti)—the one that you were born with. It's the stuff that doesn't change much—your bones, your eye color, and your general temperament. When you did your checklist earlier, your original dosha is most likely the dosha with the most checks. And then there is the out-of-balance dosha (*vikruti*), or the one that happens to be out of balance for you right now.

The original dosha you had when you were born may be the same as the one that is out of balance in you now. Or it could be totally different. In other words, by nature and birth you may be a solid kapha mountain mama with a firm, steady nature and a tendency toward unconditional love. But because of the stresses of your work, your relationship, your finances, your kids, and so on, vata gets high in your mind, and you begin to feel restless and anxious and have problems falling asleep. In this case, we would say you have kapha prakruti (meaning that you were born with a kapha nature) and vata vikruti (meaning that your current imbalance is in your vata energy).

I'll give you another personal example. By birth, I estimate that I have about 40 percent pitta, 35 percent vata and 20 percent kapha. But there was a time in my life when I really struggled with anxiety and feeling kinda out of my body. My mind was racing constantly and I felt really ungrounded. Even though my birth dosha was highest in pitta, my imbalance was clearly in vata. So which do we treat? The imbalance! Let's look at what each of these doshas is like when it is in balance and out of balance, as well as what to do to get back in balance. This will make it clearer on how you can start to bring your own imbalances back to balance.

Vata

When vata is balanced:

- Digestion is good. You eliminate on a daily basis without strain.
- You've got zest. The immune system is in an optimal state.
- You experience a longing to create, and a thirsty enthusiasm for life.
- You feel social. You want to connect with others.
- Your mind feels awake and open.
- You sleep through the night and wake feeling energized.
- Worry or anxiety may occasionally arise, but you notice it and take time to slow down.

When vata is unbalanced and needs calming:

- You feel flighty and unfocused.
- Anxiety is high.
- You get constipation and gas.
- You get sandpapery skin—dry, cracked, and rough.
- There is a lack of juiciness in your tissues, as well as life. You feel unsatisfied.

- You feel exhausted and overworked, and yet it's hard to relax.
- You may wake up around 2:00 to 4:00 AM for no apparent reason.
- It is hard to make decisions.
- You feel supersensitive and easily affected by outside events and the opinions of others.
- Because there is a lack of healthy boundaries, you may take on the burdens of others.

Note: We all experience imbalanced vata in our bodies from time to time. It manifests as pain, cramps, spasms, confusion, doubt, worry, bloating, constipation, dry skin, dry vagina, and chills.

How to calm out-of-balance vata:

- Think "warm and wet" for all life experience. Warm baths, warm stews, warming spices, and warm words of encouragement (to self and others) will melt vata's cool nature. Oiling your skin, doing things that "turn you on" sensually, taking a dip in the ocean (if the water's warm!), and putting avocado oil on your salad are ways to get more "wet."
- Reduce the amount of raw, light foods in your diet.
- Eat warm, oil-rich foods like avocados, sweet potatoes, and other "mushy" vegetables.
- Eat foods that are whole and natural but also heavy, warming, sweet, sour, and salty.
- Spice your foods.
- Take a vacation from alcohol, any form of drugs, smoking, and coffee.
- Get a good night's sleep. Give yourself the luxury of sleeping for as long as you want.
- Get on a routine of regular meditation, slow-moving yoga, and specific mealtimes.
- Be in warm environments.

- Get some loving touch, either from a friend, lover, child, or body worker. Excessive vata is reduced by touch. Use warm sesame oil, unless you think you may have a toxic system. (To learn the telltale signs of a toxic system, flip to page 72.)
- Get out in nature. Talk a long walk. Sleep outside, if it's warm enough.

Pitta

When pitta is balanced:

- Digestion is healthy. You eliminate once or twice a day and your pee doesn't burn.
- Your body doesn't suffer from inflammation.
- You have a healthy drive for life. You are motivated and face life with courage and leadership.
- Your skin isn't overly oily or suffering from acne.
- You are organized, speak clearly, and lead from a place that empowers others.
- You are not overheated or overly thirsty.
- Your mind feels clear and focused.
- You go to sleep by 10:30 PM and wake feeling refreshed.
- Anger or intensity may occasionally arise, but you notice it and can come back into balance quickly.

When pitta is unbalanced and needs cooling:

- You feel stressed or intense.
- You are overly critical, bossy, intense, or act like a perfectionist.
- You take your anger out on everyone else.
- You have loose stools, heartburn, or heat in your urine.
- Your skin is red, hot, or overly oily. You may suffer from some type of inflammation, such as burning stools, acne, or rash.
- You feel a lack of sweetness in life.
- You feel angry, impatient, or irritable.

- You stay up late—perhaps working—and can't get to bed until between midnight and 2:00 AM.

Note: We all experience imbalanced pitta in our bodies from time to time. It manifests as hyperacidity, fever, inflammation, hot flashes, soreness, anger, rage, critical nature, diarrhea or loose stools, constipation, dryness, and chills.

How to calm out-of-balance pitta:

- Think "cool and sweet" for every life experience. Take a swim in a river. Get out in fresh air. Speak and hear spontaneous "sweet nothings."
- Eat cooling foods such as mint, fennel, cucumber, coconut oil, and coconut water.
- Spice foods with cooling additions such as cumin, coriander, mint, and cardamom.
- Reduce alcohol and coffee.
- Take a moonlit walk.
- Buy roses. Put a few drops of rose essential oil on your pulse points.
- Avoid spicy hot foods, hot tubs, saunas, and hot weather.
- Put a teaspoon of fennel seeds in cool water. Drink often.
- Relax. Be spontaneous.
- Get on a routine with meals. Do not skip lunch.

Kapha

When kapha is balanced:

- Your digestion is healthy. You eliminate at least once a day and don't feel sluggish.
- Your body feels strong and your mind stable.
- You are loyal, dependable, and loving. You are able to be a support for others and yourself. You can forgive and let go.
- You have good energy reserves and immunity.

- Your skin is milky-soft and smooth.
- Your body is well lubricated.
- Your body is in optimal weight range for your height and bone structure.

When kapha is unbalanced and needs stimulation:

- You have no zest—little motivation or "get-up-and-go."
- You feel heavy or blocked in general.
- You have mucus, feel congested, or suffer from other respiratory conditions.
- You get overly sentimental, attached, or greedy. You hoard material objects.
- You get lethargic digestion and may have mucus in your stools.
- Your skin gets clammy and pale.
- You gain excess weight.
- You oversleep and feel groggy.

Note: We all experience imbalanced kapha in our bodies from time to time. It manifests as lethargy, congestion, mucus, fluid retention, joint pain, weight gain, feeling of heaviness, grogginess, overattachment, and greed.

How to stimulate out-of-balance kapha:

- Eat your heaviest meal in the middle of the day, when your digestion is strong. Eat a light dinner at night. For example, have a bowl of soup or greens with steamed vegetables. Broiled and roasted food is also great to rebalance kapha because it steams the water out.
- Add warming spices to food, such as garlic, cinnamon, onion, cayenne, leeks, and ginger.
- Do not nap during the day. Wake with the sunrise.
- Get more exercise.
- Dry brush your skin.

- Think "light and mobile" for every life experience. Be spontaneous. Take a random road trip.

• • Essential Ideas • •

- The five elements are Ether, Air, Fire, Water, and Earth.
- The elements are physical and metaphorical forces for understanding the material and energetic world, as well as the relationships between things. They are both practical and archetypal.
- Ayurveda is based on the concept of three mind-body types called doshas—or "forces that easily go out of balance."
- Vata is kinetic energy (movement). Pitta is metabolic energy (transformation). Kapha is potential energy (stability and lubrication).
- You are most likely dominant in 1–2 of these doshas. Some rare individuals have an equal amount of all three.
- Your prakruti is the doshic combination you had at birth. You will have this unique combination throughout your life. Your vikruti is the way that your dosha is out of balance currently.

Putting Ayurveda to Work

Get out your journal and answer the following: Which dosha, or mix of doshas, best describes your long-term tendencies? Which dosha seems to be imbalanced in you now?

How do you feel the force of vata in your life in both positive and negative ways? What about pitta? Kapha?

What qualities are you experiencing in your body, mind, or life right now? Do things feel rough or smooth? Hot or cool? Intense or stagnant? Light or heavy? Irregular or stable? Exciting or dull? Light or dark? Dense or clear?

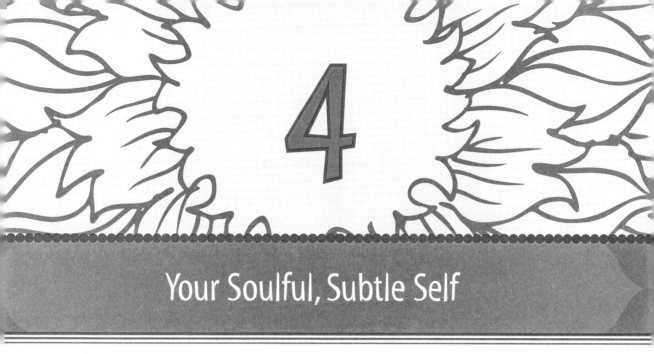

Your Soulful, Subtle Self

Now that you have started to understand the doshas, we can explore some deeper, subtler aspects of our health and well-being through Ayurveda. You may be wondering, "Okay, what happens when I start to balance my doshas? Do these forces simply go away?" Not at all. In fact, when the doshas mentioned in the previous chapter are balanced, they become our greatest allies. In this way, what was once the force behind our weaknesses can now act as a force for empowering our body, mind, and spirit, as well as enlivening our life goals.

One of Ayurveda's main teachings is that we balance our doshas, so that the subtle forces or energies that support the doshas are flowing intelligently and are empowering. Each of the doshas contain and provide an energy force: *prana*, *tejas*, and *ojas*. Prana is vata's subtle energy: it is the guiding force behind all of life's processes, our breath, and our movements. Tejas is pitta's subtle energy: it is our deep transformational ability, the light of revelation, and the warmth of personality. Ojas is kapha's subtle energy: it is related to our core immunity, mental stability, and the body's ability to renew and restore itself. These three subtle energies correspond and complement the positive, purely health-boosting aspects of the mind-body doshas of vata, pitta, and kapha. Let me explain. In the same way that our physical body is made of the materials we eat, digest, and reconfigure into muscle and skin, the subtle body is made up of sensory, energetic, and experiential material we consume and reconfigure as emotion and spirit. In other words, you are what you eat, and you are what you see and feel. If we want to understand our own subtle body, we need to take stock of all the impressions we experience through our emotions, intuition, intelligence, and spiritual connections.

Personally, I can feel the way that my own mind and body have to digest the subtle impressions I feed them. If, for example, I spend hours on the internet, getting lost in the black hole that is Pinterest or mainlining Facebook videos, I actually feel exhausted afterward—and maybe even a little sad. Whereas, if I sit outside after dinner in the moonlight and soak in the sound of Virginia crickets, after a while, I start to feel calm. My mood even turns devotional. Crickets and moonlight feed me. The internet (in excess) depletes me.

So, there are sensory impressions that feed us in a healthy way. You can come up with your own list of healthy sensory-foods. For me they are things like sunsets, Gillian Welch's music, baby giggles, tears of joy, and the smell of fresh-baked bread. Your list may be different. But the question is, from an energetic standpoint, are you eating junk food or nourishing food?

The subtle energies are not only sensory; they are also affected by the material world of food, lifestyle habits, and even weather. It is sobering to think that the news programs we watch have an effect on the health of our subtle body. And while we cannot live in a bubble, it helps to take these effects into account when we consider how we choose to spend our time.

So, just as you can profoundly affect your health by eating well, you can positively impact your subtle body through things like deep breathing, yoga, calming your senses, building powers of concentration, and good old-fashioned love. When we work to build balance with our doshas, we can then positively create these subtle energies—and we take a step closer to not only empowering our life's desires, but also understanding who we really are. Let's look at each of them in depth.

Prana—Our Guiding Intelligence

It's a miracle we have prana [PRAH-NA]. Prana is the animating, activating force that gives life to all things. It is the power behind our breath, our thoughts, our nervous system, and our emotions. While our physical body handles the mechanics of life, prana is the remarkable force that keeps our blood pumping, our heart beating, and our metabolic processes functioning optimally. Western medicine might relate to prana as the autonomous nervous system. This is the aspect of our body's intelligence that we don't have to consciously manage. For example, you don't have to plan breathing; it just happens. Ayurveda classifies prana more broadly, across many of our biological systems; it is the healing and subtle energy of vata (Air and Ether), allowing us to grow and expand our awareness. The reason why we feel better after a yoga class is because we have changed our prana. We have moved energy that may have been stuck in our shoulders from a day of working at a computer, and in this way, cleared out any minor blockages that may have built up. Energy also gets stuck when we think the same yucky thoughts, day in and day out. *Oh, I will never be able to leave this job. I will never find love. My body (finances, husband, life . . .) will never change.*

Prana can't flow smoothly through us if we are constantly multitasking, overusing technology, drinking too much caffeine, or overdoing it in general. A person with good prana has vitality, ease in their breath, good circulation, movement, and adaptability. To increase your prana, eat fresh organic foods. Overcooked restaurant foods, over-processed foods, boxed and canned foods—even "healthy" ones—are

---

Seane Corn's Five Nonnegotiables for Keeping Prana Flowing

There are five "nonnegotiables" in my own life that I rely on to keep my own prana body as healthy and flowing as possible. If these nonnegotiables are compromised in any way, I know that I am setting myself up for an energetic relapse into very familiar unhealthy patterns of shutdown. In the past, I would have leaned into these unhealthy patterns to self-medicate, using things like drugs or alcohol. But today I rely on five nonnegotiables for keeping my prana flowing smoothly: diet, yoga asana, meditation, prayer, and psychotherapy.

When these five things are consistent in my life, I feel like I am on my game physically, emotionally, and spiritually. There are just too many habits and factors in life that can pull us away from our prana, the primal life force. These five nonnegotiables keep me from being reactive. My relationships feel solid. And I don't get ill. Most importantly, they keep me from disconnecting from Source, the God of my own understanding.

(Check out her full interview on prana and feeling healthy, happy, and sexy with Seane Corn at www.healthyhappysexylife.com.)

energetically dead. They have no life force. Pranayama (the conscious guiding of energy) increases prana. Mindful movement such as yoga, tai chi, and intentional dance also liberates our energetic channels and increases optimal pranic flow through the body.

Start Now: Feeling Your Prana

Find a comfortable position and close your eyes. Take a few deep breaths. Relax for a minute, allowing your breath to deepen and smooth out. Now slowly start to draw your attention away from your thoughts, emotions, or aches and pains, and drop it down into your belly. Bring a loving awareness into your navel. The simple rule is this: Your prana follows your focus. Whatever you focus on, you move your subtle prana energy into. You may be feeling more energy in your belly. It may feel like swirling light, electricity, or benevolent honey-gold energy in your belly. You may feel nothing at all. That's okay. Remember, prana is following your focus—so if you are focused, it's working. Take a few minutes to rest in your prana, noticing how—over and over—you can shift your focus and experience your inherent guiding intelligence moving to your navel, opening you to the first subtle energy.

Tejas—The Power That Brings Out Our Light

Tejas [TAY-JUS] is the illuminating light that comes from your inner radiance. It is the healing and subtle energy of pitta. It is the fuel of transformation, the fiery essence behind all of our thoughts, and the force that brings out our light. In your body, it is the subtlest aspect of your digestion that can turn food into nourishment. It is also the energetic force behind the body's ability to see and process light. It is the glow that loving people emit. When we say, "She has a light in her eyes," it is the energy of tejas we are seeing.

Tejas is also the subtle force of the Divine living inside us that truly changes who we are. For example, we all know that the positive outcomes of a good yoga class, a retreat to the mountains, or an amazing church service are short. You leave feeling better. You leave with a shift in perspective. But how long does it last? It only takes one traffic jam, one argument with your spouse, or one hectic workday to send you right back into the old patterns of your life. Sometimes it can seem that the positive effects have gone right out the window and we quickly slip back into old mind patterns and feelings.

Tejas is the empowering force that transforms who we are. One translation of tejas is the "shininess" that is the result of being heated or burned from within—a Divine spark or flame. Think of this flame as the fire that burns your ego. This fire consumes old patterns of behavior, dissolving the mindsets that hold us back from purposeful living. Tejas experiences make us a different human being. People may experience the power of tejas when they have a near-death experience. Life itself is a sort of fire if we allow its hardships, as well as its beauty, to melt us and modify us through its lessons. When we experience tejas, there is a physical result: a resplendence and radiance of personality that draws and melts the hearts of all who come near.

A person with good tejas has radiance, a twinkle in her eyes, clarity, insight, courage, compassion, and fearlessness. You can increase your tejas through meditation, by bringing awareness to the navel (the seat of Fire), doing certain breath practices, eating a cleansing diet, and using warming, pungent spices.

Start Now: Build the Power of Your Light—Tejas

Find a comfortable position and close your eyes. Take a few deep breaths. Relax for a minute, allowing your breath to deepen and smooth out. Now, slowly start to draw your attention away from your thoughts, emotions, or aches and pains, and drop it down into your belly. Bring your awareness into your navel. Moving your attention is prana. Sustaining your focus there is tejas. Now, hold your focus on your navel. Every time a thought or emotion arises, draw your attention back to your belly.

The simple rule is this: The radiance of your tejas is the result of sustained focus. By sustaining a loving gaze, for example, you build the power of transformative fire. You boost the power that allows you to remain in the fire of life's trials and triumphs. Rest in your tejas, watching how you can stay focused and experience your inherent transformational power.

Ojas—The Power That Sustains Us

Think of ojas [OH-JUS] as the container that holds your abundant energy. It is the ultimate energy reserve of the body and mind. It is the purest essence of kapha, and physically, it is related to reproductive, hormonal, and cerebrospinal fluids. I love the metaphor of ojas as the body's natural honey; it is the delicate and refined essence we produce from the plants and other vital essences we take in. Whereas tejas is the force of our transformation, ojas is the force that enables us to sustain that change over time. Think of it as your psychophysical container or shield.

As a society, we don't respect this energy enough. The more ojas we have, the more impervious we are to illness and the negativity of others. Robust ojas acts as a soft shielding, helping us ward off stress and disease brought on by physical pathogens as well as psychic pathogens (emotional vampires, be gone!). Our own spirit has a good, strong container. Ojas gives us an overall sense of satisfaction with life. As you might suspect, our modern Western culture is chronically low in ojas.

A person with good ojas is calm and content, and has both strong immunity and endurance. This is the most important element for most of us to cultivate. Ayurvedic and yogic scholar David Frawley uses the metaphor of a light bulb to make this point: "You can think of prana as the energy going toward the light bulb, tejas as the electrical force, and ojas as the capacity of the bulb. Unless you increase the capacity of the bulb, you will always be limited, no matter how much energy is being sent to the bulb."[1]

But increasing our level of ojas is not just a matter of building it up. It is also about not losing or wasting it. When you are overstimulated, for example, if you spend hours on the internet, drinking coffee, and texting friends, you lose energy through the five senses in ways you aren't even aware of. This leaves us feeling depleted and can bring on depressive or anxious sensations. The practice of *pratyahara*, that is, controlling our senses by moderating our speech and sexual energy and getting proper rest, relaxation, and sleep, helps us preserve our vital energy. The next time you feel depleted, think of drawing the mind inward instead of reaching outward for comfort. I like to lie down and practice feeling the sensations in my body, turning my focus inward and letting any stagnant emotions rise to the surface.

Start Now: Feel a Connection to Your Ojas

This exercise will help you feel the strength of your energy reserve. Find a comfortable position and close your eyes. Take a few deep breaths. Relax for a minute, allowing your breath to deepen and smooth out. Now, slowly start to draw your attention away from your thoughts, emotions, or aches, and drop it down into your belly, holding it there until you feel sensation. Then, slowly, bring your awareness into your heart. Remember a moment in your life when you felt very deep love. Perhaps it was the birth of your child, a merging into the arms of your lover, being hugged by a parent, or the bliss you experience when you help someone in need. Maybe it was a time when you let yourself be totally vulnerable. When you add love to your point of focus, it builds your ojas.

Bring that moment fully to mind and notice where you feel the sensation of love in your body. Allow this sensation to move, expand, and permeate every cell of your being. When you grow the feeling of love inside your body, you boost the power that enables you to remain strong and wise in the face of heartache, disease, and change.

Relax into this loving container, watching how, over and over again, you will gain and lose the feeling, and how you can refocus and experience your inherent enduring and sustaining power.

• • Essential Ideas • •

- Prana is our ability to expand, circulate, and adapt to life's ever-changing landscapes. It is the positive, life-bringing force behind vata dosha. When we balance our vata, prana is energizing, giving us enthusiasm and creative potential.
- Tejas is our ability to be transformed on a deep level so that we shine. It is the positive, life-bringing force behind pitta dosha. When we balance our pitta, tejas is transformational, giving us charisma and a warmth of personality.
- Ojas is our ability to create containment. It is the positive, life-bringing force behind kapha dosha. When we balance our kapha, ojas is sustaining, giving us stability, physical immunity, and emotional well-being.

Putting Ayurveda to Work

These days, everyone needs a little more support in the realm of ojas. Here is a recipe for building and conserving your vital energy (ojas):

- **Go organic:** Eat foods that are organic, in season, and, when possible, local.
- **Cleanse and purify, then rebuild and renew:** If you are full of toxic gunk from overindulging in meat, sugar, drugs, alcohol, or processed and fried foods, don't just start eating a ton of ghee and dates! First, take a few days to eat super simple and clean foods—mainly whole grains, lentils, vegetables, and high-quality fats such as olive oil. Then, once you feel cleaned up, you can start to eat more nourishing foods such as ghee, avocado, dates, milk, and honey.

- **Avoid overeating:** This depletes your digestive fire.
- **Avoid excess stimulation while eating:** If you want to build your core vitality, don't watch the evening news during dinner or eat lunch in front of your computer.
- **Rest:** Sleeping 8 hours at night is paramount for building ojas. Rest also means taking a break from constant "doing" to relax and deeply unwind. Turn to page 114 for an overview of Ayurvedic sleep routines.
- **Oil your outer body:** Chapter 9 of this book will teach you how to use oils, as well as which oils may be best for you in terms of body temperature and seasons.
- **Oil your inner body:** Yes, that's right. Drinking and eating more oils boosts ojas. Incorporate more oils such as hemp, flax, avocado, coconut, and ghee into your diet.
- **Say no to vampires:** Avoid the people, places, and media that disturb your mind or suck your soul blood.
- **Spend more time in nature**
- **Rest your mind:** See chapter 12 for how-to's.
- **Do *nasya*:** See page 129 for how-to's.
- **Do restorative yoga:** Most yoga studios have a "restorative" class. If not, check this book's resources section for some how-to's.
- **Love the one you're with:** Any form of genuine love and devotion boosts your core vitality and immune system.

Things that will sap your core vitality:

- Travel (especially in airplanes)
- Overexercising
- Serious physical injury
- Letting yourself get excessively hungry
- Overanalysis, overthinking, and any form of mental disturbance like doubt, lack of faith, anger, greed, or jealousy
- Unprocessed anger, worry, anxiety, or grief

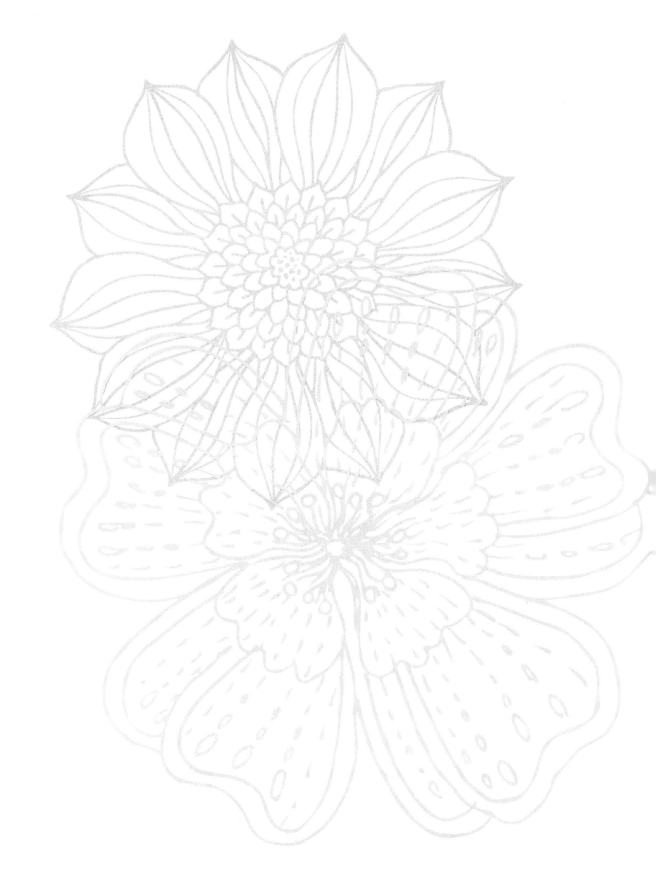

Part II

Healthy

*A*yurveda says that food is prana (energy), and that all beings are in a constant search for more. Your own prana is created by the life you take from food. Plants, animals, and minerals make a sacrifice for you, and hopefully you are using them to become more self-aware and more loving. In this way, step one of Ayurvedic nutrition is to clean the lens of perception from one of mindless consumption, to one of deep gratitude for the sacrifice.

We become more powerful when we eat loving, home-cooked, fresh food. Somehow, in the context of modern culture, it has become a luxury for us to cook for ourselves and loved ones. Our great grandparents took it as a given that making meals was a part of life. With the advent of pre-prepared and processed foods, as well as the explosion of fast food, sometimes cooking for ourselves takes a backseat to our busy lives. I believe that much of the modern health malaise in our society parallels this lost relationship. But there is nothing that shows your commitment to health more—and there is nothing sexier—than a woman or a man who knows how to cook.

This doesn't mean that we have to quit our job and spend hours in the kitchen. I really believe that you can change your health (and your destiny), by spending as little as 30-45 minutes in the kitchen daily. Cooking for yourself will dramatically alter the way you feel within your body and mind, as well as create a healthier body for tapping into your soul. Creating beautiful, whole-food meals will give you increased energy, better mood, healthy weight levels, and more radiant skin with reduced wrinkles and inflammation, as well as a clearer mind.

This practice isn't just about cooking for ourselves. It's also about learning to be self-aware. This means stopping your life, putting your hand on your heart, breathing deeply, and asking your body, "Body, what do you *really* need?" Self-awareness is the most crucial element of good health—and this is the cornerstone of Ayurvedic wisdom. By bringing loving self-awareness to the choices we make around food, we are better able to hear our body's response to what we put into it—as well as reduce our susceptibility to pathogens and disease. Every morsel of food or drink that we take in has the capacity to be a healing nectar or a toxic bomb. Usually, if we practice self-awareness, our own wise body will help us discern nectar from toxins.

In my experience, when I am eating a whole-food, nourishing diet on a daily basis, I make better decisions in regard to how I spend my time. If I eat fried, processed, and sugar-laden foods, made by non-loving, nonbreathing food-processing machines, I feel a lack of love in my belly. This lack of love reduces my ability to be my most authentic self in the world. Simply stated, we are *what* and *how* we eat. If we eat in a hurry, our body feels rushed and anxious. If we eat crap, we feel like crap. If we eat brightly colored organic veggies, we feel brightly colored, full of energy, and organic to our true nature. From the basis of self-awareness and a recognition that food is one of the key ways we build our energy, we can now deepen into the energetic and elemental qualities of food.

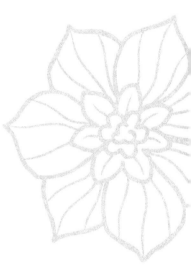

My Own Evolution toward Healthy

I remember being a chubby thirteen-year-old girl and holding Susan Powter's *Stop the Insanity* diet plan in my hands. It felt like a promise. If Susan could go from being morbidly obese to a lean, mean, diet-business queen, I could stop eating peanut butter sandwiches in bed at night. Now don't get me wrong; I think Susan's success is amazing, and many diet plans are directed at helping people get out of their suffering—but what these results-focused diets don't do is teach us how to access the root of our healthiness. As a plump teenager, I didn't learn how to really listen to my body or how to nurture it. I learned to come at food from a place of intellectualization (think counting calories) and self-hate (think "No, you can't have cake, fatty!").

Ayurveda helped me (and continues to help me) heal this disconnection between my inner knowingness (that truly senses what food I need) and my internal dialogue (that can shift from being a drill sergeant to an overly indulgent parent). When I learned Ayurveda, I learned a Nature-loving, time-tested framework for understanding food energetically. I also learned what foods are best at what times of day and year. Ayurveda also taught me how to combine foods in the best ways, so as to kindle my digestive fire.

Philosophically, I learned that food is sacred. In fact, Ayurveda says food is a form of God. And when you treat food like God, the whole landscape of your relationship to food shifts. The act of eating is also a divine transformation, whereby food goes from being an apple into becoming you! And you are also a form of God. In this way, truly radiant health is built upon taking the time to recognize yourself and the food you eat as manifestations of the Divine. Most importantly, Ayurveda taught me how to access the part of me that can *deeply* listen to what my body needs. I can't wait for this chapter to deeply feed you. I hope that you kindle that kindhearted voice between your body's needs and the foods you bring to it. I know that this is the start of the healthiest life possible.

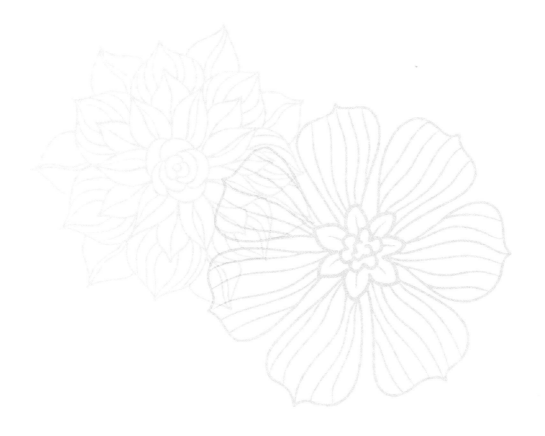

5

Ayurvedic Nutrition and Your Dosha

Ayurvedic nutrition is built upon the doshic view of the universe. Remember back to chapter 3 when we looked at the concept of your original mind/body constitution at birth (prakruti), as well as the dosha that is out of balance in your now (vikruti). These two may be the same, and they may be different. The more you know about your vikruti (your current imbalance), the more you can tailor your diet to that imbalance and start feeling better.

Imagine, for example, that you are a pitta type by nature, but you have been really run down for the past few days. Your skin feels drier than normal, you have been experiencing constipation, some insomnia around 2:00 to 4:00 AM, and a certain amount of anxiety. Each of these are vata expressions, meaning they increase the qualities of dry, cool, and mobile in you. In this instance, it would be a

good idea to reduce vata by eating in a way that is the opposite of dry, cool, and mobile. Therefore, your food needs to be unctuous, warm, and slightly heavy. Opposites balance each other, so by paying attention to the language of the body, we can make tuned-in food choices.

I have also found that when people are healthy and have good digestion, any doshic type will benefit from eating seasonally, just as Mama Nature intended. That said, if you have a dosha that is out of balance, switching over to the food list that reduces that dosha can be immensely helpful. Remember, these are general guidelines, and Ayurveda is highly individualistic. Nothing takes the place of meeting with an Ayurvedic practitioner to deeply explore your personal constitutional imbalances and to create a food program that will address your needs. Check out the

"Ayurvedic Education Institutions" in the resources section of this book if you are looking for a qualified practitioner.

The Seasonal/Doshic Food List

Everyone can eat from the vata-reducing list if it is fall/early winter and they are healthy. You may also choose to eat from this list any time you need warming, grounding, stabilizing, comforting, or wetness in your body. This list can be medicinal for most people who have vata disturbances such as jetlag, gas, belching, dry skin, constipation, and anxiety. Foods listed as "Best" can be eaten daily. Foods listed as "Small amounts" can be eaten a few times a week. Foods listed as "Avoid" should be eaten only on special occasions.

The Healthy Fall/Early Winter List—Reduces Vata

Basic idea: Increase the sweet, salty, and sour tastes.
Avoid: Bitter, astringent, and pungent tastes

Grains

It is best to eat these as cooked grains.

Best: Amaranth, oats (cooked), quinoa, basmati rice (white or brown), unprocessed wheat
Small amounts: Barley, millet
Avoid: Buckwheat, corn flour (chips, bread, and tortillas), dry oats (granola), polenta, rye

Dairy

Best: Butter, buttermilk, kefir, milk, sour cream, cottage cheese or queso fresco, yogurt (fresh)
Small amounts: Hard smelly cheese
Avoid: Ice cream, frozen yogurt

Sweeteners

With vata, moderation is key. Even the healthiest form of sweets can cause imbalance in excess.

Best: Raw, uncooked honey, maple syrup, molasses, brown rice syrup, Sucanat

Small amounts: Date sugar

Avoid: Brown sugar, white sugar

Oils

Best: Almond, ghee, sesame

Small amounts: Avocado, castor, coconut, flaxseed, mustard, olive, peanut, sunflower

Avoid: Safflower

Fruits

Best: Baked apples, apricots, avocados, bananas (ripe), black-berries, cantaloupe, cherries, coconut, cranberry sauce, fresh dates (not dry), figs (fresh), grapefruit, grapes, lemons, mangos, nectarines, oranges, papaya, peaches, pears, persimmons, pine-apple, plums, raspberries, strawberries (ripe), tangerines

Small amounts: Apples (sour is best), pomegranate

Avoid: Dried fruit of any kind, cranberries

Vegetables

Cooked vegetables are best. Most raw veggies will disturb vata.

Best: Avocado, beets, carrots (not as a juice), leeks, mustard greens, okra, onions (well cooked), parsnips, shallots, acorn squash, winter squash, sweet potatoes, tomatoes, water chestnuts

Small amounts: Broccoli, cauliflower, celery, corn, cucumber, eggplant, green beans, kale, medium chilies and hot peppers, mushrooms, potatoes, radishes, seaweed, spinach, sweet peas,

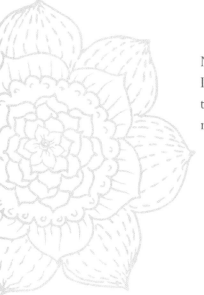

zucchini. Lettuce, spinach, and any leafy green can be eaten uncooked with a creamy or oily dressing occasionally.

Avoid: Alfalfa sprouts, artichokes (unless served with a butter-lemon sauce), asparagus, bean sprouts, brussels sprouts, cabbage (even cooked), raw vegetables, snow peas

Nuts and Seeds

Nuts should also be eaten in moderation, and lightly roasted and salted. Dry roasting should be avoided. Nut butters are fine. Remember, in the past, nuts were a special treat to be sprinkled on dishes. Nuts are not a meal!

Best: Almonds

Small amounts: Cashews, hazelnuts, pecans, piñon, pistachios, pumpkin seeds, sesame seeds, sunflower seeds, and any other nut not mentioned

Avoid: Peanuts

Meats

If you choose to eat meat, limit consumption to 2–3 times per week. Meat soups can be particularly nourishing when you are depleted, fatigued, or overcoming sickness. If you are depleted, meat-broth stews are particularly healing.

Best: Beef, chicken and turkey (dark meat), duck, eggs, freshwater fish, lamb, pork, seafood, venison

Small amounts: Chicken and turkey (white meat), shellfish

Legumes

Best: Mung beans

Small amounts: Tofu, hummus

Avoid: Aduki beans, black beans, chickpeas, fava beans, kidney beans, lentils, Mexican beans, navy beans, pinto beans, soybeans (except as tofu or soy milk)

Spices

Best: Anise, basil, bay leaf, caraway, cardamom, catnip, cinnamon, clove, cumin, dill, fennel, fenugreek, garlic, ginger (fresh), marjoram, mustard, nutmeg, oregano, pepper, peppermint, poppy seeds, rosemary, saffron, sage, spearmint, thyme, turmeric

Small amounts: Cayenne pepper, cilantro, ginger (dry), horseradish, mustard, parsley

Avoid: Any spices in excess as this dries out tissues

Condiments

Best: Mayonnaise, vinegar

Small amounts: Ketchup

Avoid: Carob, chocolate

Beverages

Best: Warm water, spicy teas such as chamomile, cinnamon, clove, and ginger

Small amounts: Diluted fruit juices (half water)

Avoid: All alcohol, black tea, carbonated mineral water, coffee, fruit juices, soft drinks

The Healthy Summer List—Reduces Pitta

Everyone can eat from the pitta-reducing list if it is summer and they are healthy. You may also choose to eat from this list when you need more cooling, drying, grounding, spaciousness in your body. This list is a medicine for most people who suffer from inflammation, hyperacidity, anger, intensity, overheated body, loose stools, acne, skin rash, or other pitta conditions.

Basic idea: Increase the sweet, bitter, and astringent tastes.

Avoid: Pungent (hot), sour, salty tastes

Grains

It is best to eat these grains cooked.

Best: Barley, white basmati rice, millet, oats, white rice, unprocessed whole wheat

Small amounts: Brown rice

Avoid: Buckwheat, corn flour

Dairy

Best: Unsalted butter, cottage cheese, cream cheese, ghee, milk

Small amounts: Hard unsalted cheeses

Avoid: Buttermilk, salted cheeses, sour cream, kefir, cultured milks, yogurt

Sweeteners

Best: Maple syrup, rice syrup

Small amounts: Honey

Avoid: Molasses, raw sugar, white sugar

Oils

Best: Ghee, olive

Small amounts: Avocado, canola, corn, coconut, soy, sunflower

Avoid: Almond, castor, flaxseed, margarine, mustard, peanut, safflower, sesame

Fruits

Best: Apples, avocados, blackberries, blueberries, cantaloupe, coconut, cranberries, dates, dried fruit, figs, grapes, lemons, limes, nectarines, pineapple, prunes, raisins, raspberries, strawberries

Small amounts: Apricots, bananas (very ripe only), cherries, grapefruit, oranges, pineapple

Avoid: All sour fruits, such as sour oranges (mandarin), sour pineapple, sour plums, papaya, olives, tangerines, and all unripe fruit

Vegetables

Vegetables should be eaten cooked in the winter. But pitta types can get away with eating them raw in the summer. Fresh green vegetable juices are also good for pitta.

Best: Alfalfa sprouts, artichoke, asparagus, bean sprouts, bell peppers, bitter melon, broccoli, brussels sprouts, cabbage, cauliflower, celery, cilantro, cress, cucumber, green peppers, kale, leafy greens, lettuce, mushrooms, onions (well cooked), peas, pumpkin, seaweed, squash, zucchini

Small amounts: Avocado, beets, carrots, corn, eggplant, garlic (well cooked), parsley, potatoes, spinach, sweet potatoes, vine-ripened tomatoes

Avoid: Chilies, hot peppers, mustard greens, onion (raw), radishes, tomato paste, tomato sauce, and any hot or pungent vegetable

Nuts and Seeds

Best: Coconut, sunflower, pumpkin seeds
Small amounts: Pine nuts, sesame seeds
Avoid: Almonds, brazil nuts, cashews, hazelnuts, macadamia nuts, pecans, pistachios, peanuts, and any other nut not mentioned

Meats

If you choose to eat meat, limit consumption to 2–3 times per week.

Best: Chicken, egg whites, freshwater fish (trout), turkey
Small amounts: Beef, duck, egg yolk, lamb, pork, sea fish, venison, any other red meat

Legumes

Best: Black lentils, chickpeas, mung beans, split peas, soybeans (soy products), tofu

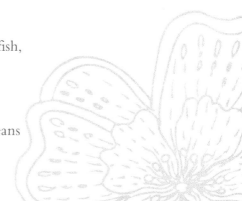

Small amounts: Aduki beans, kidney beans, navy beans, pinto beans

Avoid: Red and yellow lentils

Spices

Best: Cardamom, chamomile, coconut, coriander, dill, fennel, lemon verbena, peppermint, saffron, spearmint, turmeric

Small amounts: Basil, bay leaf, black pepper, caraway, cinnamon, cumin, ginger (fresh), oregano, rosemary, thyme

Avoid: Anise, asafetida, calamus, cayenne pepper, cloves, fenugreek, garlic (raw), ginger (dry), horseradish, hyssop, marjoram, mustard seeds, nutmeg, poppy seeds, sage, star anise

Condiments

Best: Carob sweetened with the best sweeteners noted above

Small amounts: Mayonnaise, sweet mustards

Avoid: Chocolate, salt, vinegar

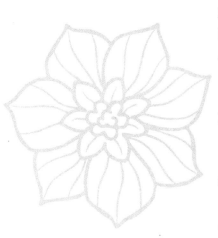

Beverages

Best: Water, milk, coconut milk, coconut water, bitter and astringent herb teas such as alfalfa, chicory, dandelion, hibiscus, and strawberry leaf, wheatgrass, and other green juices

Small amounts: Chai tea or black tea, fruit juice diluted by half with water

Avoid: Alcohol, carbonated water, coffee, sweet fruit juices, spicy herb teas, soft drinks, tomato juice

The Healthy Late-Winter/Spring List—Reduces Kapha

Everyone can eat from the kapha-reducing list if it is spring and they are healthy. You may also eat from this list when you need more dryness, lightness, and circulation in your body. This list is a medicine most people use as a remedy for mucous conditions, excess weight, and fluid retention or heaviness in digestive system.

Basic idea: Increase the pungent, bitter, and astringent tastes.

Avoid: Sweet, sour, and salty tastes

Grains

Toasted breads are very good for kapha, as they are drying.

Best: Amaranth, barley, basmati rice, buckwheat, corn flour, quinoa

Small amounts: Millet, rye

Avoid: Oats, long- and short-grain rice (white or brown), wheat, whole wheat

Dairy

Best: Goat's milk, skim milk, soymilk

Avoid: Butter, buttermilk, cheese, cream, cottage cheese, ice cream, kefir, sour cream, yogurt

Sweeteners

Best: Raw honey only (in moderation)

Avoid: Fructose, maple syrup, molasses, raw sugar, white and brown sugar

Oils

Use all oils in small amounts only. Even the best oils, if overused, will aggravate kapha.

Best: Canola, corn, flaxseed, mustard, safflower, soy, sunflower

Avoid: Almond, avocado, castor, coconut, olive, peanut, sesame

Fruits

Best: Dried fruits, apples, cherries, cranberries, grapefruit, pomegranate, prunes, raisins

Small amounts: Apricots, lemon, lime, papaya, pineapple

Avoid: Sweet fruits, avocado, bananas, berries (raspberry, blackberry, blueberry, strawberry), cantaloupe, coconut, dates, figs, grapes, mango, melons, pineapple, oranges, peaches, pears, persimmons, plums, tangerines, watermelon

Vegetables

Vegetables are best eaten raw during the summer and cooked the rest of the year. Sometimes kapha individuals may find that raw foods dampen their digestion and need to be avoided completely.

Best: Alfalfa sprouts, artichoke, asparagus, green beans, bell peppers, broccoli, brussels sprouts, cabbage, cauliflower, carrots, celery, chilies, cilantro, corn, kale, lettuce and other leafy greens, mustard greens, onions, parsley, peas, hot peppers, potatoes, radish, seaweed, spinach, rutabagas/turnips

Small amounts: Beets, cucumber, eggplant, mushrooms, okra, squash (all), sweet potatoes, tomatoes, water chestnuts, zucchini

Nuts and Seeds

Best: Pumpkin seeds, sunflower seeds

Small amounts: Sesame seeds

Avoid: Almonds, brazil nuts, cashews, coconut, hazelnuts, lotus seeds, macadamia nuts, pecans, pistachios, peanuts, walnuts

Meats

If you choose to eat meat, limit consumption to 2–3 times per week. Kapha individuals can thrive as vegetarians more than pitta or vata doshas.

Best: Chicken or turkey, freshwater fish, rabbit

Small amounts: Eggs

Avoid: Beef, duck, lamb, pork, seafood, shellfish, venison

Legumes

Best: Mung beans, red lentils, soybeans (tofu and soymilk), split peas

Small amounts: Aduki beans, black beans, black gram, fava beans, kidney beans, lima beans, pinto beans

Avoid: Black lentils, chickpeas

Spices

Best: Anise, basil, bay leaf, black pepper, calamus, chamomile, caraway, cardamom, catnip, cayenne, cinnamon, cloves, coriander, cumin, dill, fennel, fenugreek, garlic, ginger, horseradish, hyssop, marjoram, mustard, nutmeg, oregano, peppermint, poppy seeds, rosemary, saffron, sage, spearmint, star anise, thyme, turmeric. Hot spices are best. Any spice not listed is probably fine.

Avoid: Salt

Condiments

Small amounts: Ketchup, vinegar

Avoid: Mayonnaise, salt

Beverages

Best: Herbal teas (spicy and bitter), cranberry juice, green vegetable juices, wheatgrass juice

Small amounts: Carbonated mineral water, coffee, tea

Avoid: Apple juice, carrot juice, orange juice, soft drinks

Remember, food is prana, so no matter what you're eating, it is providing your energy, your life force. When we don't pay attention to our bodies and eat whatever we crave (whether it's junk or simply hot sauce when we're already too fiery), it can affect our energy. This is why most people can eat from the seasonal lists if they are healthy and aren't experiencing imbalances, digestive or otherwise; nature is providing for us and telling us that if we're in balance, this is what will provide us with the best energy. If you are having some health issues (digestive problems or other minor health imbalances) working to reduce the dosha that's bugging you through diet can have a profound impact on your wellness. In fact, when we adjust diet, oftentimes medicine (both herbal and pharmaceutical) is no longer needed.

• • Essential Ideas • •

- Ayurveda holds that food is prana; what we eat directly affects our energy, our life force.
- When we are reasonably healthy and have good digestion, we can eat seasonally, partaking of what Mother Nature is providing.
- When we feel ill or are dealing with belly woes, we can eat from the dosha-reducing food list that is appropriate for our imbalance.

Putting Ayurveda to Work

- What season is it? If you feel great, have fun going to the farmers' market or grocery store and shopping from your seasonal list. You can also download and print my seasonal list from my website: www.healthyhappysexylife.com.
- Start simply. If you do feel out-of-whack, take a moment to write down any health complaints or imbalances in your digestive system. Determine which dosha is giving you trouble.
- Have gas, bloating, or constipation? Print up the vata-reducing list and go shopping this week. Have the intention to eat as much from the vata-reducing foods as possible. Have loose stools, heartburn, or a generally "heated" feeling? Go shopping with the pitta-reducing list. Are you retaining water, excess weight, or feeling full of mucus? Go shopping with the kapha-reducing list.
- Check out appendix A (page 223) for seasonal menu planning ideas and recipes.

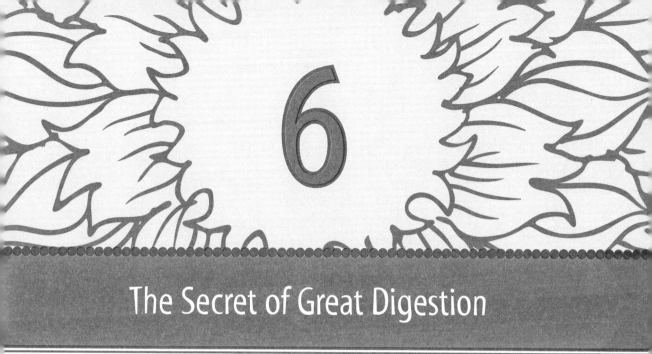

6

The Secret of Great Digestion

If you want to feel vital and beautiful, the dietary secret is universal:

Good Digestion +
Good Assimilation/Absorption +
Good Elimination =
Feeling Like a Bombshell

Being an Ayurveda bombshell isn't about the way you look. Being a bombshell is about how you feel. We all know that eating the right foods is essential for a beautiful body, good skin, a clear mind, and energetic balance. What we may not be aware of is that healthy eating is not enough. The best food on the planet can't help you if you don't have the digestive fire to transform and assimilate what you are putting in your body. The ancient texts called this digestive fire *agni*. Agni is what transforms and assimilates what we are taking in, whether it is food, life experiences, or thoughts.

Ayurveda holds that many of our diseases start with the accumulation of toxins (ama) in the body. This sludge builds up when our metabolic fire is unable to burn what we are putting into the body. Our metabolism slows down, or gets dampened, when we throw junk food on our fire. If you drink a lot of ice water, you are dampening your fire. If you eat a lot of processed food, leftovers, or canned and frozen foods, you dampen your fire. And whatever is not cleanly digested hangs around in the system and forms a sludge. With time, this sludge gets harder and harder to move. This is why we do cleanses. Cleanses help move ama. If you notice you have a few of these symptoms, and they tend to be chronic, it may be a sign that your metabolic fire is weak.

Twenty-one signs you may have a dampened metabolic fire (agni):

1. Unexplained weight gain
2. Belly bloat
3. Burping or gas
4. Acidity or heartburn
5. Itchy rectum
6. Loose stools or constipation
7. The feeling that your poos just aren't "complete"
8. Feeling super full after a normal-sized meal (or that you need a post-meal nap)
9. Nausea
10. Acne
11. Dry, cracked nails
12. Dry, cracking skin
13. Parasites
14. Bad breath
15. Lots of coating on tongue
16. Allergies
17. Candida
18. PMS (premenstrual syndrome)
19. Eczema, hives, and other rashes
20. Psoriasis
21. Unexplained brain fog, bad mood, lethargy

How Did I Get Toxic Sludge Buildup?

Life is fast and oftentimes we are stressed, hungry, and reaching for whatever food is in sight just so we can make it to the end of the day. Bad food choices, negative thinking, stress, and a fast-paced lifestyle lead to digestive imbalances. With time, micro-imbalances lead to macro-imbalances and you are left with ama, a rotten by-product of bad digestion. When this sludge builds up, it prevents our belly from getting the good nutrients out of the healthy food we are eating. Ayurveda views ama as the single most toxic threat to our radiant health.

Getting rid of ama is like doing a body-temple sweep that cleans out physical toxins, as well as old emotion- and mind-states. By cleaning up the belly, you will also clear out long-stored emotions and thought patterns in the body. Boosting your digestion and getting a perfect poo can lead to the following radical health boosters: better immune function, cleared sinuses, clearer skin, better sex drive, more energy, less excess belly fat, less burp-fart-burp-itis, mental clarity, calmer nerves, and, of course, poophoria. And how do we do this? By paying attention to what we put into our bodies.

Start Now: Simple Ways to Lessen Toxicity and Boost Your Belly Fire

Eat light at night. Soups and milky/spicy herbal teas at night make the belly happy and help us detox.

Ginger, freshly sliced. Squirt a lemon on it and add a pinch of salt. Eat a few slices before and/or with meals to boost metabolism and gut enzymes.

Drink milk alone or with things that are sweet (such as grains, honey, brown sugar). Milk digests best when it is hot and spiced.

Get to know these superstar medicinal spices: turmeric, ginger, cinnamon, cardamom, nutmeg, cumin, coriander, fennel, and black pepper.

Getting the Perfect Poo (Yeah, I said it . . .)

A lot of Ayurvedic nutrition is about getting the perfect poo. If you walk down the aisles of any drugstore in this country, you will see a testament to our collective indigestion. From antacids to stool softeners, we take for granted how unnatural it is to need a pill to help our body release its toxic waste. Here again, we can call in the ancient wisdom of Ayurveda, which believes in the reflection of the macrocosm in every microcosm, even our individual poos. As the Earth herself shows us her ever-increasing inability to digest the toxic overload of the landfills and chemical pollutants we throw onto her body, why are we surprised when we suffer from very similar imbalances, such as constipation, increased intolerance, and sensitivities to foods? Whatever happens to Mama Earth is gonna happen to her children. Modern research supports ancient Ayurveda's understanding of the importance of daily bowel health.

Truly, physical health or imbalance can be traced back to the quality of our elimination. It's hard to feel happy (much less reach enlightenment) when we aren't having what I call "poophoria," or the contentment that comes from having a wonderful poo on a regular basis.

You may currently feel so disconnected from your poo that you don't know that poophoria feels like. How often should it happen? What should it look like? When I ask women, "So, how is your elimination?" some immediately giggle nervously and answer, "Oh, it's normal." But what is normal? "Normal" for some of us means having a bowel movement (BM) once every three days! Or one day having tough, dry stools and the next day diarrhea. This is not poophoria.

In the perfect world of delectable poos, we would be going to the bathroom once a day. If we have a more pitta constitution, we may go twice a day. Normally, this should occur in the morning, without the need for a laxative. Normal poos do not require a cup of coffee to get things moving. After your morning motions, you should feel light, energetic, and that the evacuation has been complete. You shouldn't feel strained or hurried during your elimination rituals. There should be no burning, gas, smells other than a food-like odor, and most definitely no pain. In essence, your morning poo should be something you look forward to, because it feels good.

The ideal poo should also be solid but soft, well built and minimally smelly. Your poos should look similar every morning, regardless of what you ate the night before. If sinkage occurs, it only happens over time, not immediately. The perfect poo is easy to wipe, does not stick to the toilet, and is brown color, like a tanned banana that smiles up at you.

What If My Poo Is Less Than Perfect?

If your poo doesn't fit these guidelines, then, well, you are out of the Ayurveda Club. Just kidding. Remember, Ayurveda is not about being perfect. It is about building loving awareness. It is also about consciously altering the conditions in your body so that Nature responds favorably. If you see that your poo has remnants of yesterday's meal, it may mean that your digestion and assimilation powers are not able to handle all the food you are throwing at it. It may also mean that what you're eating is not agreeable to your constitution or the seasons. It may mean your emotions are a little unprocessed or you are mentally stressed. The more you use and learn the principles from this book, the more your poo will magically respond.

Simple tips for the perfect poo:

- Drink more ginger tea. Fresh ginger is best.
- Eat more oils (i.e., flax, hemp, fish oil).
- Check in with your poos. Avoid the foods that you see showing up undigested.
- Follow the doshic and seasonal guidelines, as well as the general rules for food combining in this book.
- Spice up your meals. Doshic-appropriate spices are our poo's best friends.
- Stop the graze-fest. In general, snacking on foods before the last snack has been digested leads to sinking, toxic poos.
- Eat freshly prepared foods. Leftovers lead to less-than-perfect poo.
- Eat fiber-rich foods to improve stool quality.
- Say "yum," and mean it. When we love what we are eating, when it smells and looks good, our bodies are listening and we digest better. Eat while sad or angry, and you can see the emotion in the "motion."

- Watch what you do while not eating. It blew my mind to find out that energy-wasting habits, seemingly unrelated to mealtimes, also dampen agni, the metabolic fire. Gossiping, watching the news or gossip-loving TV talk shows, engaging in arguments, talking for the sake of filling the silence, or obsessively checking email are all examples of agni killers.

Food Rituals

Ancient Ayurveda honored food through prayer and ritual, as it encouraged human beings to be in a place of gratitude when involved in consumption. If you think about it, it's a miracle that food (something that is not you) can be eaten and will become a part of you. Ritualizing the eating process brings you into a connection with the Spirit, in both your food and yourself. By praying or lovingly ritualizing your food, you reduce any neuroticism you hold around food. Taking time to say a blessing also changes your mindset to a more positive one before you eat, which betters your digestion and assimilation capacities.

Easy ways to ritualize food:

- **Offer gratitude.** Give thanks to Big Mama Nature's food. Feel that She is providing you with nourishment through the sacrifice of other plants and animals.
- **Set the table, even if you are eating alone.** Laying down a beautiful tablecloth, placemats, and cloth napkins tells your unconscious, "Eating is sacred."
- **Feed someone else first.** In Ayurveda, we first feed others as a sign of our gratitude to the Big Mama who is feeding us. If you are single, make some extra food for a neighbor, water the plants, or feed the birds.
- **Focus on the food.** Eating while web-surfing, watching TV, texting, or driving dampens the digestive fire.
- **Chew slowly and mindfully.** Feel grateful for where you are now in your life.

- **Eat in a good mood.** Our mood carries power into the food we eat. If we eat while we are angry or sad, or any other negative mood state, that mood will be transmitted into the food we eat, and deeper into the body and mind.

Simple Secrets for Great Metabolism

Now that you've put some power of ritual into your relationship with food, let's explore the ways to boost, or at least balance, your metabolism. Pick 1–2 things on this list to really incorporate, so as not to overwhelm yourself. When those feel like second nature, start incorporating a few more.

- Drink a cup of warm lemon water first thing in the morning. About one quarter of a medium-sized lemon in a normal coffee cup full of water will suffice.
- Avoid breads, pastries, cookies, cakes, all fried foods, cheese, canned and processed foods, leftovers, nuts, alcohol, sugar, and pasta.
- Eat your main meal at lunch. This is when your metabolic fire is strongest!
- Eat dinner around 6:00 PM. Eat a light dinner of steamed veggies, rice, and/or a warm bowl of soup.
- Cook with spices that boost digestion: dried or fresh ginger, fennel, black pepper, cayenne, mint, rock salt, cinnamon, nutmeg, cardamom, dill, turmeric, cumin, coriander, and ajwan seeds. These spices not only help us digest and absorb, they also help pull toxic sludge out of the system.
- Avoid snacking between meals.
- Eat a thin slice of fresh ginger before meals. Add a pinch of rock salt and a spray of fresh lemon or lime juice.
- Eat only until three-quarters full.
- Don't ever (ever, ever) drink ice water with meals. Avoid drinking large quantities of liquid with your meals. Why would you throw ice and lots of water on a fire?

- Drizzle ¼ teaspoon of olive oil or ghee (clarified butter) on your meal before eating it.
- When using grains, nuts, seeds, lentils, and rice, it's best to soak them at least 30 minutes before cooking. Some harder beans may be soaked overnight. Cook them with spices such as ginger, black pepper, asafetida, or even a little seaweed. These spices help prevent gas and bloating, and make them easier to digest.
- Throw out your white table salt. It is full of poisons—chemicals that leach nutrition out of your bones. Only use real, unprocessed salts like sea salt and Himalayan rock salt.
- Drink more digestive teas like ginger, cardamom, fennel, cumin, and coriander.
- Drink ¼ cup of organic aloe vera juice in the morning and in the evening before bed. This is highly purifying and helps boost the body's ability to assimilate the nutrients in food.
- Consider taking ½–1 teaspoon of triphala powder before bed (see the resources section on where to buy). This fruit-based powder scrapes the intestines of sludge. It also helps restore proper peristaltic action in the bowels.
- Do a simple *kitchari* cleanse with a qualified Ayurvedic practitioner.
- Eat more of these metabolism-boosting foods: soups, most spices, garlic, leafy greens, olive oil, limes, oatmeal, apples, pears, grapefruit, green tea, tomatoes, broccoli, celery, parsley, nettles, turmeric, beets, fennel, carrots, fresh ginger, and mung beans.
- Avoid these, always and forever: anything that says "low fat," "no fat," or "sugar free." The natural fats and sugars in these foods have usually been replaced with love-killing chemicals. Eliminate white sugar and table salt; all chemically treated, genetically modified, hormone-pumped, chemically fed, chemically preserved or processed, irradiated foods; artificial sweeteners and colorants; food fried in old oils; trans fats; and fat substitutes like margarine and shortening.

- Go organic! Not only do pesticides and GMO-modified foods dampen digestion, they have also been shown to cause nervous system imbalances, neurological deficits, cancer, hormonal disruption, severe and moderate mental imbalances, ADHD (attention deficit hyperactivity disorder) and endocrine system disorders.

Love-Your-Belly Food Combining

Different foods require different digestive enzymes to break them down. Throwing two foods with dramatically different enzymatic requirements at your body is like yelling at your belly, "Hey, you, work harder!" By avoiding these sad-belly food combinations, we make life easy for our poor little tummy, and it can respond by giving us great digestion and amazing glowy-ness.

Here's the deal:

1. Eating fruit alone is best. Melon should always be eaten alone.
2. Milk should be taken alone or with things that are sweet (grains, honey, brown sugar, etc.) Milk digests best when it is hot and spiced. Great milk spices include: cardamom, cinnamon, turmeric, black pepper, and nutmeg. Milk has a particularly hard time alongside bananas, sour fruits, yeasty breads, fish/meat, and yogurt.
3. Avoid eating any dairy products with fish.
4. Eggs don't mix well with fruit, milk, meat, and yogurt.
5. Honey should never be boiled or cooked. Mix it with ghee in equal amounts (by weight).
6. Nightshades (eggplant, tomatoes, potatoes) don't mix well with melon, cucumber, or dairy.[1]

Start Now: From Fire to Nourishment

In this chapter, we have been discussing ways to boost agni—your metabolic fire. Once this fire is balanced, you can begin to rebuild and strengthen your whole body. How do you know your agni is balanced? Your tongue will look clean and rosy. You will start to feel "hungry" at regular times during the day. And you will have less of the gnarly toxic-buildup symptoms mentioned in this chapter. With less toxic buildup, your body can now handle slightly heavier, more nourishing foods that increase core vitality. When we have strong core vitality, we can better ward off stress and disease. These foods will help you not only endure life, but thrive.

- Sesame seeds and sesame oil
- Pumpkin seeds
- Dates
- Coconut and coconut oil
- Avocado and avocado oil
- Olive oil
- Bee pollen
- Oats
- Barley
- Almonds (soaked in water overnight, skins removed)
- Flax seeds and flax oil
- Walnuts and walnut oil
- Raw honey
- Raw organic cow or goat's milk/cream
- Ghee or butter
- Sweet potatoes and yams
- Okra
- Squash
- Eggplant
- Spinach
- Mango
- Raisins
- Blueberries
- Mung beans
- Red lentils

- Homemade buttermilk
- Homemade unsalted cheese
- Bone broth and stews

• • Essential Ideas • •

- Good Digestion + Good Assimilation/Absorption + Good Elimination = You feel healthy, happy, and sexy.
- When and how you eat are as important as what you eat.
- Ayurveda says that food combining is as important as eating "healthy foods."
- It's not enough to just eat "healthy" foods. You must have the digestive fire (agni) to assimilate nutrients and eliminate waste.

Putting Ayurveda to Work

- Look back at the lists in this chapter. Do you have any signs of dampened agni?
- List three ways you are going to implement radiant belly-fire health techniques this week or month.
- Make a grocery list of core-vitality-boosting foods to add to your diet this week. Here are some basic pantry must-haves. If you are new to whole foods, head to the store and buy these ingredients. You'll have a lot of fun playing with them:
  - Ghee
  - Coconut oil
  - Lentils
  - Mung beans
  - Rice (my favorite brand is Lotus Foods Organic Rice)
  - Oats
  - Quinoa
  - Lemons
  - Ginger
  - Other fresh fruits and seasonal vegetables

– Seeds (such as pumpkin, sesame, sunflower, and so forth)
– Nuts (almonds are a must . . .)
– Spices
– Herbal teas

This week, pay close attention to your digestion. Keep an ongoing food journal of what and when you ate. Notice how you felt during the meal. What was your mood? How did your belly feel directly after the meal? Were you light or lethargic? Note any symptoms. How did you feel an hour or so after the meal?

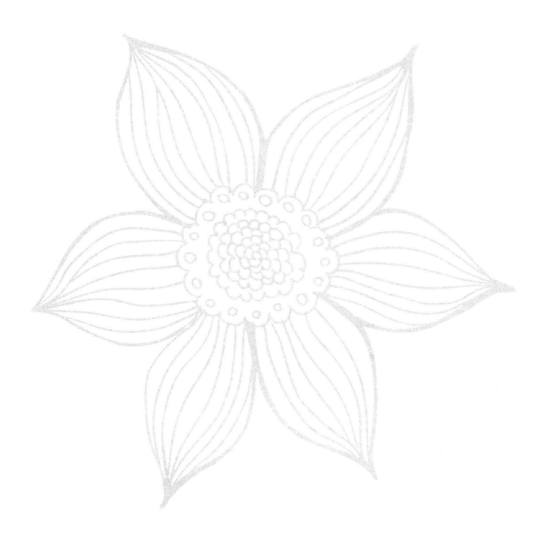

Food and the Emotions

At this point in our study of Ayurveda, it will come as no surprise to hear that food deeply affects your mind and emotions. The beauty of this science lies in its time-tested, deep study and categorization of foods and herbs into tastes (*rasas*). We can work with different tastes and other subtle qualities to balance cravings and free ourselves from the emotion/food struggles that so many of us face.

The Sap of Life Has Six Flavors

Ayurveda divides the tastes into six categories: sweet, salty, sour, pungent, bitter, and astringent. The goal is to get a little of all six tastes into your meals (unless you are working with a specific imbalance or disease). When we are healthy, making each meal an expression of the six tastes leads to profoundly positive physical, psychological, and emotional effects.

When we skip some of the tastes, we typically get the feeling that something is missing, even if our belly feels full. We should learn to trust this feeling of lack. It is a clear indicator that, indeed, one or more of the six tastes was absent. Sadly, the Standard American Diet (SAD) is mostly sweet and salty. The SAD actually lacks the very tastes (bitter, pungent, astringent) that would quell our society's chronic inflammatory imbalances and obesity.

Our life experiences also hold distinct rasas. Pay attention to how different relationships leave you with a particular flavor. Some interactions feel sweet and grounding. Others may leave a bitter taste in your mouth. See if you can notice whether certain experiences leave you craving a particular food. If you don't feel sexually satisfied, you may reach for candy, ice cream, or wine for quelling your need for warm, sweet-tasting sexual nourishment. Or you may feel unfulfilled in your career. Because of this lack of filling, you may reach for heavier tasting foods that fill up an empty space. And sweet and heavy aren't necessarily "bad." In fact, each have a medicinal value for both the body and the mind, in the proper amounts and at the right time.

Here is a more detailed breakdown of the energetics of the six tastes. Please, do not get overly analytical with the idea of the tastes. You will begin to incorporate the tastes into meals intuitively with time. In general, the sweet taste should be the bulk of the meal (e.g., rice, whole grains, some types of veggies). And the other tastes will come through in smaller amounts.

The Six Tastes[1]

Sweet

Qualities: Heavy, cool, moist, wet

Doshic effect: Increases kapha, reduces pitta

Examples: Grains, breads, rice, honey, sugar, meat, milk, most
fats, most fruits, nuts

Benefits: Builds tissues; rejuvenates and nourishes us; hydrates,
tones our muscles; softens and builds the skin, hair, and voice;
boosts longevity; soothes us; grounds us; strengthens us; com-
forts us; connects us; reassures us; and heals us

With the right amount of the sweet taste, we feel satisfied and grounded. Too much leads to feeling fat and swollen, having clogged pores, oily skin, congestion, lethargy, cystic acne, pus, blackheads, and puffiness in the face and may even result in diabetes, strong cravings, greed, and depression.

Sour

Qualities: Heavy, hot, warm, oily

Doshic effect: Increases pitta and kapha, reduces vata

Examples: Vinegar, sour apples, raspberries, tempeh, yogurt, fermented foods, citrus fruits

Benefits: Cleanses skin, boosts metabolic activity, digestion, adds firmness/strength to tissues, stimulates sweating, gets rid of gas and bloating, improves elimination, increases appetite and salivation, moistens food we eat, creates alertness and sharpness in the mind

With the right amount of the sour taste, we feel sharp, clear, and ready for action. Too much leads to envy, jealousy, and a "soured" disposition, excess thirst, muscle weakness, loose stools, dark circles under eyes, hyperacidity, anemia, dizziness, lifeless skin, acid reflux, ulcers, and other burning sensations.

Salty

Qualities: Heavy, hot, moist

Doshic effect: Increases pitta and kapha, reduces vata

Examples: All salts (rock salt, sea salt), seaweed, seafood

Benefits: Boosts digestion, opens blocked channels, improves circulation, softens organs as well as lumps and tumors, decreases general stiffness, increases saliva, is a mild sedative and laxative, awakens mind, strengthens heart, creates a sense of enthusiasm, builds courage

With the right amount of the salty taste, we feel fearless and courageous. Too much leads to water retention, contraction, itching, wrinkles, weight gain, inflammation, debility, thirst, high blood pressure, acidity, chronic feeling of dissatisfaction, burning, swollen glands, skin discoloration, premature aging, balding, and greed.

Pungent

Qualities: Drying, light, hot

Doshic effect: Increases pitta, reduces vata when taken in small amounts, reduces kapha

Examples: All spicy peppers and chilies, ginger, garlic, basil, cardamom, cinnamon, cloves, mustard, horseradish, oregano, rosemary, thyme, spearmint

Benefits: Boosts appetite and digestion, opens blocked channels, improves circulation, purifies food, promotes sweating, relieves nerve pain, gives skin a glowing quality, aids in weight loss, helps dissolve fat and toxins, kills parasites, moves blood stagnation

With the right amount of the pungent taste, we feel a lust for living life; we're passionate, clear, and excited about the direction we are taking. Too much leads to burning sensations of all types, warm skin, inflammation, dryness, broken capillaries, increased blood pressure, ulcers, acidity, heartburn, dry skin, dry lungs, loose stools, jealousy, anger, lust and passion, weakening of our fertility, and even emaciation.

Bitter

Qualities: Drying, light, cool

Doshic effect: Increases vata, reduces pitta and kapha

Examples: Leafy greens, green tea, mate

Benefits: Powerfully antibacterial, germicidal antiviral and anti-parasitical, used to detoxify the body, reduce tissues, purify the blood, promote weight loss, create tightness in the skin and muscles, used as a fat scraper, tonifier, and cleanser for the organs

With the right amount of the bitter taste, we feel clear in the mind and toned in the body. Too much leads to anemia, low blood pressure, and a feeling of being ungrounded and "airy." This can lead to anxiety, isolation, grief, and fatigue, as well as physical depletion. Too much of the bitter taste can overly reduce our tissues, leading to dryness, constipation, dehydration, premature wrinkles, chills, vertigo, and compromised immunity.

Astringent

Qualities: Drying, heavy, cool

Doshic effect: Increases vata, reduces pitta and kapha

Examples: Most lentils and beans (including green beans), green apples, pomegranate, cranberries, açaí berries, asparagus, teas high in tannins

Benefits: Antiseptic, constricts channels that are overly open, holds nutrients in the body, shrinks pores, controls excess sweating, removes mucus, helps heal sores and wounds, reduces inflammation and cools, slows or stops bleeding and diarrhea

With the right amount of the astringent taste, we feel grounded, safe, and focused. Too much leads to dryness, gas, constipation, contraction, close-mindedness, insecurity, nerve pain, and general irritability. Our life options seem limited; the mind feels scattered and fearful. Too much astringency can also lead to intestinal cramping, spastic colon, premature aging, and weakness or stiffness in the body.

Working with the Six Tastes

Just being aware of our need for all six categories of taste will be a powerful way to start feeling more fulfilled. Ideally, a balanced meal would include all of the six tastes, although you might want to adjust the quantity of the tastes for your own dosha. For example, a kapha person should use a little less of the sweet taste while a vata and pitta would benefit from using more if it. We may also want to reduce a particular taste that may be harmful to us at a particular time. For example, the pungent taste (spicy) would be harmful for anybody, regardless of their dosha, if they are suffering from burning indigestion. Similarly, the bitter and astringent tastes are not helpful if we are constipated or have vaginal dryness. This is why I recommend that people who suffer from vata issues, such as constipation, anxiety, or dry skin, not eat bitter leafy greens or drink green smoothies. These are the tastes that will actually make them feel worse. In general, a moderate amount of all six tastes will be beneficial for everyone. It's only when we become addicted to one or more tastes that imbalances happen.

So, how do we work with the tastes when trying to become more balanced in our dosha? Try not to overcomplicate things initially. Work with balancing the doshas as per the instructions from the dosha chapter, and you will naturally be consuming more of the tastes you need and less of the tastes you don't. Read over the qualities of the tastes and start to identify any specific imbalances you may suffer from, avoiding those tastes that may really harm your current condition. For example, as stated above, the astringent taste is very drying (increasing to vata dosha). So, if you know that you are struggling with chronic dry skin, avoiding super-astringent foods like açaí berry, green apples, and lentils is a good idea. Then, when things feel more balanced, you can come back to enjoying a little of all six tastes, while emphasizing vata-reducing foods that are sweet, heavy, and moist.

Emotional Eating

Have you ever noticed that admitting you are an emotional eater, overeater, or unconscious eater is a somewhat embarrassing admission? Geneen Roth starts her book *Women Food and God* with the following bold assertion: "The way you eat is inseparable from your core beliefs about being alive. Your relationship with food is an exact mirror of your feelings about love, fear, anger, meaning, transformation, and, yes, even God." *Oh my*, I thought. If that was true, then I was not being present with God at all. In fact, I ate in a distracted, rushed way, ignoring God completely. And then there was the emotional eating. Indeed, it was amazing to watch the direct relationship between unprocessed fear or grief and potato chip purchasing.

Food, in essence, is the energy of Mother Nature. When used appropriately, it is an amazing gift for feeling grounded and nourished. And in many ways, we are forced to find a balanced relationship with food. Unlike alcohol, drugs, or even sex, where an addict can swear off the problematic substance for all eternity, food is an essential. Without it, we die. In this sense, food is simultaneously our connection to that which is greater than our individual bodies and souls, as well as our first essential desire to be nourished by our Earth Mother.

Ayurveda understands imbalance in our cravings as a consequence of misunderstanding. Because of the nourishing nature of food, we overindulge in an attempt to feel secure, safe, and loved. And it goes even deeper than this. Ayurveda says that if, when we were little girls, our natural cravings were not honored, then we probably created some unnatural patterns of desire, instead of listening to the innate wisdom of the body. Think about it. Did anyone actually teach you to listen to your body? To ask your body, *What do you really need?* The tastes and cravings we developed as girls have a way of persisting into our adult lives. If we were taught healthy food habits, chances are we still have them. Similarly, if we were fed sweets for being a "good girl," or admonished for eating fattening foods, chances are we will tend toward imbalance.

Digestive imbalances in our bellies, whether they be gas, constipation, heartburn, or other forms of indigestion, are our belly's call-out for love. Our tummies may be angry or anxious because of our own lack of self-care. Or they may just be wisely showing us where we are feeling some anxiety or upset in the mind. Belly imbalances don't just come from overconsumption of junk food. Even if we eat super-healthy food, if we eat too much, or if the digestive fire is not strong or if we eat when sad, stressed, or angry, the body bears the burden. That's why when I am going through a rough patch mentally or emotionally, I start making kitchari or vegetable soup.

Unhealthy cravings speak to what is lacking in our life experience. But how can we know the difference between healthy and unhealthy cravings? When a healthy desire is fulfilled, we feel uplifted and expanded. When we fulfill a healthy food craving, we feel energized and alive after we eat it. Unhealthy food cravings temporarily fulfill an emotional need, but make us feel off in our body later. We can look at our unhealthy taste cravings for insight into what we may be lacking, consciously or unconsciously, in the realm of our emotional needs.

Meditation on Feeding the Goddess Within

Prepare for this meditation by choosing your ritual food object. It can be as simple as a tangerine, or as complex as a tiramasu. Bring this food into your meditation space. Now, close your eyes and gently turn to your breath. Feel your belly relax, your jaw soften. After your mind settles, imagine that inside of your heart exists a radiant little Inner Goddess. You can visualize her as the most beautiful creature you have ever seen. See her clearly in your mind. Sitting in the cave of your heart, she waits in hungry anticipation for what you will feed her. Imagine what you would offer to her. In what way would you prepare the food? What foods would you choose to offer this perfect being? What would the table setting look like? Would there be candles or lights? Music playing? How would you present this meal to her? Imagine how she would consume the fare. Would she rush or take her time? See her in your mind's eye. After the meal, does she rush off to her next meeting, or does she rest in your heart, allowing herself time to assimilate what you have so lovingly given to her? Now, take your ritual food object in hand. As you place this object in your mouth, see her in your body. As you taste the food, feel that she is tasting it. Continue to enjoy your treat as if you were ritually feeding this inner Divine One. Come back to this meditation anytime you feel rushed, distracted, or that you are emotionally eating. Notice how this act affects your mind and your digestion.

The sweet taste is like the "cuddling" of food. Sweets are the quintessential go-to-taste for getting our emotional needs met. Why? Because emotionally, when we taste something sweet, we experience a moment of feeling nourished. In healthy amounts, it also brings softness and stability to mind and body. So, imagine the end of a hectic, stressful day. Maybe no one hugged you or reassured you. No one touched your skin and told you, "Hey, everything is gonna be okay, lady." In this scenario, it makes sense that the emotional body would reach for sweets to make you feel nourished and safe. To reduce sweet cravings, we must go into the deeper issues of our own life. And the question we can ask ourselves is, "Where in my own life am I lacking deep nourishment, softness, and stability? How can I change that?"

Emotionally, the sour taste makes us feel warm and grounded. Wine is a great example of a sour (and sweet!) go-to craving. From an Ayurvedic perspective, we love wine because it relaxes us, dilates the blood vessels, and makes us feel earthy. The sour element also focuses the mind. We may crave the sour tastes when we don't feel grounded and focused in our life. Too much of this craving leads us to become sour in our countenance. Think sour grapes.

The salty taste allows us to retain. If our life feels scattered and our energy feels dispersed, we may reach for this taste. If we feel like we are constantly giving but not holding in, we may go for the salty taste. When we emotionally crave saltiness, we may also lack confidence and enthusiasm for life, as this taste offers us those sensations in healthy amounts. The downside is that no amount of salt can boost our confidence for long. In excess amounts, salt creates feelings of greed. If you crave this taste, ask yourself, *Am I giving out too much? How can I build my own self-worth and enthusiasm for life?*

The pungent taste causes the blood to circulate and the heart rate to increase. In balanced amounts, pungent tastes such as ginger and black pepper help boost circulation and cleanse the body. But when we crave this hot taste for emotional reasons, we may be reaching for its capacity to temporarily induce feelings of pleasure, excitement, and courage. If you constantly crave hot, spicy foods, ask yourself, *Is my life boring me? Am I afraid to ask for the excitement I really want in my life?*

It is less common to crave the bitter taste for emotional reasons. Usually, when we crave the bitter taste, it's because our body is asking for something that can dry up and scrape away excess fat and moisture. The bitter taste is highly purifying, and it asks the ego (which loves the sweet taste) to temporarily give up its pleasure. If you do feel like you have an unhealthy craving for the bitter taste, it may be a sign of self-denial. If we are overly concerned with self-control, or are overly attached to overcoming our ego, we may start to use this taste in unhealthy ways.

The astringent taste is another, more rare emotional craving, but it can occur. Emotionally, the astringent taste temporarily offers the sensation of drawing in. It causes our body to become dryer and colder. Unhealthy cravings for too much of this taste could be a sign of the desire to withdraw from one's life. While this taste temporarily enables us to collect our thoughts and withdraw from the world, too much can create unwarranted fear of opening up.

Unconscious Craving to the Super Mama's Pleasure-Power

So, how can we really know the difference between the desires that are healthy (*satyakama*) and the desires that want the temporary emotional fix but leave us longing for more (*asatyakama*)? The answer to the delicate relationship between women, emotion, and food lies in moving from the unconscious to the conscious. This means that when we feel the urge to overindulge in any of the tastes, we call in the big guns. We call in the Super Mama. Who is she? She is the part of you that lovingly winks at the patterns of your old cravings, and she caresses that scared little girl who feels that her belly needs to be overly full in order to feel the earth beneath her. She is also the loving mama, living inside of you, that asks the hyper-controlling aspect of yourself to be in the pleasure of eating.

The first stage in bringing the darkness of unbalanced craving into the light is to identify it. Write it down. Admit the way you feel a dysfunction or disconnection from your pleasure-power in regard to food. Secondly, as the disconnection arises, see it as an opportunity for bringing light into unconsciousness. Put your hand on your heart and say to yourself, *My darling, what do you really want?* Thirdly, try to cook for yourself or eat food from hands that have lovingly prepared it. Remember, your soul is seeking love and connection. Just filling your belly will not satisfy this deeper pleasure. Also, trust your direct experience in regard to digestion and satiety over any recent pop-science study, and especially over the advertising you see on TV or in the news. When you fall back into the realm of poor consumption choices, pull this book off your shelf, go to the recipes section, and start cooking up some inspiration. Lastly, there are no hard-and-fast laws in this book. Do not believe anything you read, but deeply commit to trying things out. Learn from your own experience. In this way, infinite possibilities for transformation occur.

• • Essential Ideas • •

- Ayurveda divides nature's tastes into six categories: sweet, salty, sour, pungent, bitter, and astringent.
- We crave certain tastes for their power to affect us mentally, emotionally, and physically. When we are balanced, we will crave tastes that bring us into more balance. When we are imbalanced,

we will crave the tastes that may offer a temporary, emotional "fix," but that leave us craving more.

- Our ability to cultivate self-awareness around how food is fulfilling unmet emotional needs will empower us to make choices for our long-term healthy, happy, sexy selves.

Putting Ayurveda to Work

Which of the six tastes do you crave the most of? Do you notice an emotional correlation with what the taste "provides"? For example, if you crave sweets, do you feel a lack of sweetness in your life? If you only crave bitter or astringent flavors, are you preventing yourself from being deeply nourished?

Choose a ritual food for your "Feeding the Goddess Within" meditation. Write down your experience from the meditation in your journal.

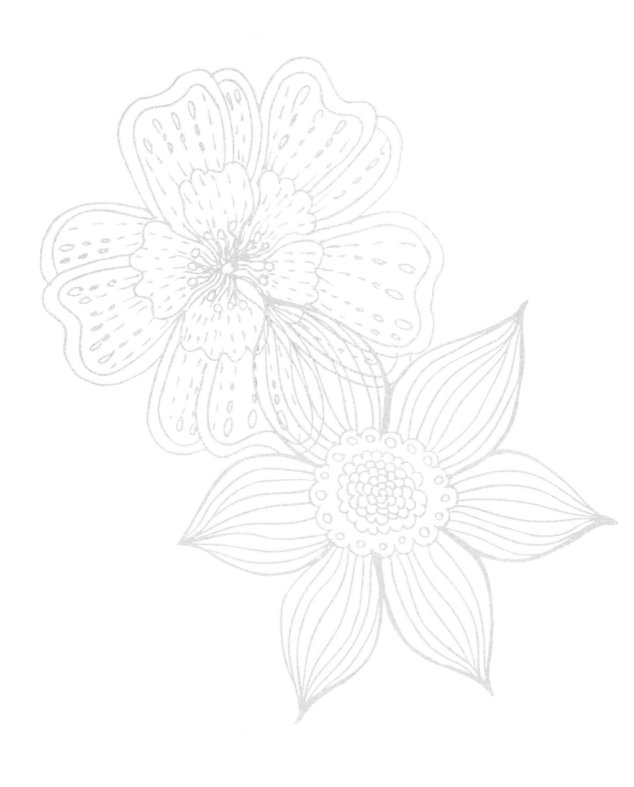

8

Setting Up a Living, Sexy Kitchen

The Dalai Lama once said, "Western women will change the world."[1] I believe him. Nicole Daedone, founder of One Taste, a cool organization that teaches people how to hold space for female sexuality, went on to elaborate on the Dalai Lama's quote, stating that it will be "turned-on women that change the world."[2] I agree. I also think that when the women of the world realize that a part of their raw, sexual, creative power can be ignited through feeding themselves and others, the consciousness of the world will shift. In fact, the single most powerful way you can improve your health is to start chopping vegetables on a daily basis.

Why? Because McDonald's food equals McDonald's consciousness, and pure, local, loving-mama, old-school food equals pure, loving, earth-abundant consciousness. Let me repeat. Eat crappy processed food and you will

feel the profit-motivated, loveless, bottom-line intentions of the makers of that food. Eat what your grandma made, and you may just get a tiny taste of not only her love for you, but perhaps what turned her on—and that is a radical, juicy-woman idea.

A Turned-On Kitchen

Let's learn how to set up a living, loving kitchen. A living kitchen pulsates with the rhythms of a woman's life. A living kitchen burns brightly when we blend up a new dressing or taste a pungent virgin olive oil. The air in a living kitchen actually tastes good, still spiced from last night's creation. Plants inhabit this kitchen, breathing moist newness into the nooks and crannies of shelves and cupboards. A wooden cutting board is stained magenta from chopping beets whose brightness now belongs to the inside of a child's belly. This living kitchen is a sacred space—a hearth and a temple where we have the potential to create the nourishment that supports life within us and for others. It is an altar to the mundane, corporeal, visceral body that radiates light and power. There is no room more powerful in a home than a turned-on woman's kitchen.

Fun fact: architecture statistics show that more family activities are taking place in kitchens, "as they are regaining their role as 'control center' of the home."[3] Could it be that these rooms are taking on a revival of importance in our modern world as a symbol of our collective need to be deeply nourished? Is this, perhaps, a revival of the hearth? The healing community fire? I hope so.

Getting your kitchen Ayurveda-friendly is not complicated, but it may be a good idea to begin incorporating new spices and buying cookware, little by little. For most of us, learning happens over time. What is more, these are my suggestions for setting up a kitchen, not rules set in stone. Most of the tools on the list may already be in your kitchen. Most of the spices are easy to find at grocery stores; the more obscure ones are available online.

Another concern that many people face when trying to live a more Ayurvedic lifestyle is the time constraints of down-home, old-school, real-deal cooking. It may help to slowly begin to shift your mindset surrounding cooking for yourself and your family. Many women already feel overwhelmed with the amount of tasks they have on their shoulders. Ask them to cook fresh veggies and soups every night, and they are likely to look at you like you are crazy. But what if we began to slowly breathe life into a living kitchen, making it a priority to reserve 30-45 minutes each morning and evening to cook for ourselves?

It is my experience and belief that this psychological shift creates a change in behavior. Seeing fresh food as a life essential, instead of a luxury for the time-rich, is key. In addition, the more we can cook for ourselves, the more energy we will have. Fresh food has more prana. Many women report actually feeling like they have more time when they cook for themselves because they suffer from less exhaustion. Start cooking for yourself and you will have more time, because you have more vibrant life breathing into you. I promise.

Also, it's a good idea to start thinking of your spice rack, refrigerator, and pantry as your own home pharmacy. You may also find that if you have kids, they begin to take interest in what you are doing if it seems like you are having fun going to the farmers' market, tasting seasonal veggies, smelling fresh herbs, playing with colorful foods, and generally being alive and sensual in your kitchen. In my experience working with moms, I have found that over and over, kids will take awhile to adjust to new foods, but with time they will actually begin to crave healthy foods. And you will too.

Before we start breaking out the cast iron, here are seven suggestions on how to bring out your Inner Kitchen Diva:

1. **Be playful.** Do not hesitate to douse your kids in flour if they need a "kitchen-can-be-fun" lesson.

2. **Experiment.** Don't start from the fear that you can't make yummy vittles. Trust your intuition. Use recipes (including the ones in here!), but don't be afraid to put down your measuring spoons and improvise. Ancient Vedic mamas cooked in *anjalis,* or handfuls. Our grandmas used bushels, dashes, pecks, and pinches.

3. **Buy a really sexy apron.** They do exist.

4. **Play some music.** If you are in a bad mood in the kitchen, music will shift the energy.

5. **Be a creatrix.** Make the food beautiful. Serve it on banana leaves. Plant edible flowers in your organic garden and throw them on your salads and rice dishes.

6. **Enlist help.** Just because this book is attempting to help women fall back in love with food does not mean we are the only ones doing the cooking. Today's world requires that all family members help out—man, woman, and child.

7. **Fall in love first.** People love their mothers' or grandmothers' food is because it is made with love, and with the loved one in mind during the process. The bottom line is that your

mood goes in the food. If you are angry at your loved ones, stop, breathe, and begin again. If all else fails and you are still upset, put down the knife and order a pizza. Seriously.

Creating a Living Kitchen— The Basic Kitchen Tools

Cooking is so much easier when you have the right tools at your disposal. Setting up a simple Ayurvedic kitchen will help you get organized in your efforts. Also, the Ayurvedic mama is hip to using modern technologies like food processors and blenders as long as they don't suck too much life out of her foods (microwaves destroy a certain amount of prana and lack the transformational capacities of real fire).

- **Electric grinder or mortar and pestle:** Used for grinding spices, nuts, seeds, and grains. I use my electric coffee grinder to grind harder nuts and grains, and the mortar and pestle for softer spices. There is a healing property we receive by inhaling the essences of freshly ground spices.
- **Food processor:** Choose glass over plastic, when possible.
- **Blender:** The Vitamix is worth the cost.
- **Handheld immersion blender for soups**
- **Nonreactive cookware:** The best materials for tapping into nature while cooking are unglazed clay, cast iron, stainless steel, copper, enamel, glass, ceramic, stone, and wood. Nonstick pans are less than ideal, but useful for sticky situations.
- **Knives:** A kitchen goddess carries a sharp sword. That's why sharp knives are a key element in any vital-woman's kitchen. Chopping and slicing can be a pleasure or a pain, according to sharpness of your knife. Invest in a high-quality set.
- **Spoons and such:** Again, try to avoid plastics. I love wooden spoons. A large soup ladle, metal spatula, slotted spoon, and whisk are a must.
- **Garlic press:** A nice shortcut.

- **Large metal grater:** Choose one with a good handle.
- **Lemon press:** The glass variety is best. Look for one that has ridges to grip the fruit better.
- **Fine grater:** For zesting lemon peel and finely grating nutmeg or hard cheeses. Look for a stainless steel brand.
- **Y-shaped vegetable peeler:** This type of peeler helps you peel tougher skins like papayas and butternut squash.
- **Peppermill:** Fresh ground pepper has more prana than other varieties.
- **Salad spinner:** Not only does it help you clean your greens, but it's great for getting rid of the excess water.
- **Wire mesh colanders:** Buy one with a foot at the bottom to ensure your pasta won't sit in the residual puddle in the sink. In a pinch you can use a small one as a flour sifter.
- **Slow cooker:** While slow cookers increase the heaviness of foods, they can be a lifesaver for the new mama or the 9–5 gal. Use the slow cooker for making ghee, and cooking lentils, soups, and stews. The best feeling in the world is to set your slow cooker on low, and wake up to toasted ghee or steamy soups the next morning.
- **Rice cooker:** Another wonderful tool for busy women. Pop the rice into the cooker, place some cooked veggies on the steamer tray, and press the button. You will have a healthy meal that you can spice and oil as needed.

Tips for Your Living Kitchen

Buy in bulk. Dry grains such as pasta, rice, lentils, and beans can be purchased in bulk and stored in glass containers. Not only do they look beautiful in their little glass homes, but it's also much cheaper and saves you the hassle of having to buy small amounts week after week.

Create a kitchen shrine. I have found that creating a small kitchen shrine reminds me of the sacred connection between my body, soul, and the food that is being prepared. Furthermore, if the energy of the cook is of seminal importance to the quality of the meal, having a small shrine helps me bring my scattered brain back into the present moment—the slice of the knife into the blood orange, the smell of the cumin seeds popping in the hot oil, the delectable feel of a ripe mango in my hand. A shrine is an external reminder of the sacred inside us. Place things on the shrine that will remind you of what you need—a small statue, a photo of your teacher or mentors, fresh flowers—anything beautiful that speaks to your heart.

Spices Are Medicine

Your wild-woman world will shift when you become a goddess of the spice. Spices are plant medicines that enhance digestion, help us assimilate what we eat, and remove toxic buildup. The harder a food is to digest, the more we need the help of spices. Even if the healthiest of foods are not spiced properly, they can produce toxic ama—even many so-called super-foods. That may be why I hated cabbage as a kid. My mom would boil it, throw some salt on it, and say, "Enjoy!" Yuck. We need to spice veggies.

Also, there is something delightful about establishing a relationship to your spices. And if you think about it, spices are pretty sexy. They are the refined aspect of the most aromatic, concentrated essence of plants. From pungent to sweet to just plain stinky, spices are extracted from bark, buds, fruit, roots, seeds, or stems of Mother Nature's own medicine cabinet. In Ayurvedic cooking, spices aren't just something we add for flavor or color, but are one of the primary ways a mama takes care of her clan. They are revered as daily doses of potent healing medicines. And today, modern science is confirming what the ancients knew instinctively. It wouldn't be a stretch to ask: Is the lack of spice in the bland American meat-and-potatoes diet leading to the onslaught of chronic conditions?

When you learn more about what herbs and spices like turmeric, cinnamon, oregano, and cardamom can do for your overall health, you will be astounded that you weren't working them into every meal, every day. Experiment. Make mistakes. Let your turmeric-stained towels be the new testament to your body's brightness.

There are hundreds of different spices to choose from. Here are some of my favorites, including their energetic properties and healing potentials:

Spice Name	Taste	Quality	Superpower	Effect on Dosha
Anise	Pungent	Heating	Light, detoxifying, boosts digestive fire	-V, +P, -K
Allspice	Pungent	Heating	Boosts digestive fire, liquefies kapha	-V, +P, -K
Basil	Astringent	Warming	Stimulating	-V, +P, -K
Black pepper	Pungent	Heating	Promotes circulation, boosts digestion, reduces kapha in respiratory system	-V, +P, +K
Bay leaf	Pungent, bitter	Heating	Boosts digestive fire	-V, +P, -K
Caraway	Sour, pungent	Warming	Reduces gas, relieves water retention/ bloating	+V, +P, -K
Cardamom	Sweet, mildly pungent	Cooling	Curbs sweets cravings, cleanses mucus, relieves gas, boosts fat metabolism	-V, -P, -K
Cayenne	Pungent	Heating	Strong circulatory, heating and drying	-V, +P, -K
Cinnamon	Sweet, mildly pungent	Warming	Boosts blood circulation, detoxifying, antiseptic	-V, -/+P, -K
Clove	Pungent	Heating	Light, antibacterial, remedy for mucus in colds	-V, +P, -K

continued on page 102

Spice Name	Taste	Quality	Superpower	Effect on Dosha
Coriander	Astringent	Cooling	Cools tissues, boosts digestion, relieves gas	-V, -P, -K
Cumin	Slightly pungent, bitter	Warming	Strong digestive, boosts appetite, cleanses fat and toxins, antimicrobial	-V, -P, -K
Fennel	Sweet	Cooling	Cooling digestive, breath sweetner	-V, -P, -K
Fenugreek	Pungent, bitter	Warming	Boosts digestive fire, promotes skin health	-V, +P, -K
Garlic	Pungent	Heating	Strong medicinal, antiparasitical, good for cold/flu	-V, -P, -K
Ginger, fresh	Pungent	Warming	Adaptogen, strong digestive, boosts agni, reduces ama	-V, -P, -K
Mint	Sweet and slightly pungent	Cooling	Boosts digestive fire, curbs cravings, antibacterial, reduces inflammation	-V, -P, -K
Mustard seed	Pungent	Heating	Boosts digestive fire	-V, +P, -K
Oregano	Slightly pungent	Warming	Boosts digestive fire, diuretic, diaphoretic	-V, -P, -K
Parsley	Astringent, pungent	Warming	Drying, reduces water retention without causing electrolyte loss, reduces flatulence, strongly detoxifying, aids in weight loss	-V, -/+P, -K

continued on page 103

Spice Name	Taste	Quality	Superpower	Effect on Dosha
Rose	Sweet, mildly bitter	Cooling	Soothes inflammation, calms nerves, tonifies the reproductive system	-V, -P, -K
Rosemary	Pungent	Heating	Great natural cure for flatulence	-V, +P, -K
Thyme	Pungent	Heating	Reduces mucus, astringent antibiotic, antiinflammatory	-V, +P, -K
Turmeric	Bitter	Heating	Digestive, antiinflammatory, cleansing	-V, -P, -K
Saffron	Astringent, bitter	Cooling	Aphrodisiac, ojas-enhancing, antidepressant	-V, -P, -K

General Smarts on Using Spices:

- **Seeds:** Seeds such as mustard, cumin, and coriander are more resilient to heat. Because of their hard outer shells, it's a good idea to sauté seeds in a little ghee or olive oil.
- **Fresh herbs:** Herbs such as cilantro, parsley, or mint are heat-sensitive and should be finely chopped and used as a garnish once food has been cooked, or should only be added at the end of the cooking process.
- **Powders:** By far the most common form of spices, powders can generally be lightly sautéed in oil but are more often simmered directly into grains, veggies, or beans as they cook. Spice powders can also be added directly to milks, dressings, or breakfast grains.
- **Barks, roots, and tougher seeds:** Perhaps the least common form of spice, barks and roots require more fire for releasing their medicinal capacities. Whole cinnamon sticks or cardamom pods, for example, can be boiled in water to release their aromas.

- **Adding to oils:** It is usually best to sauté spices (and salt) in an oil such as ghee or coconut oil, as it allows the medicinal properties of the spice to be released and more efficiently carried to the seven *dhatus* (tissues). In fact, Ayurveda considers oils to be "carriers" for medicines. In this sense, the body can better absorb the spice.

Churnas: Spice Blends to Have on Hand

What I love about *churnas* (spice blends) is that I don't have to worry about adding 5–6 different spices to my meals. You can add 1–2 teaspoons of these spices to soups, stir-frys, sauces, or grains. Sauté them in a little oil until the aroma is released.

Vata-Reducing Spice Mix
- 2 tablespoons whole cumin seeds
- 2 tablespoons whole coriander seeds
- ½ teaspoon cardamom seeds
- 1 teaspoon licorice powder
- 1 tablespoon ginger powder
- 1 tablespoon turmeric powder
- ¼ teaspoon asafetida (hing) powder
- ¼ teaspoon Himalayan sea salt

Note: You can also play with adding a little black pepper, raw sugar, fennel seeds, mango powder, or star anise.

Pitta-Reducing Spice Mix
- 2 tablespoons whole fennel seeds
- 2 tablespoons whole coriander seeds
- 2 tablespoons whole cumin seeds
- 1 tablespoon whole cardamom seeds
- 2 tablespoons chopped dried mint leaves

- ¼ teaspoon ginger powder
- 1 teaspoon licorice powder

Kapha-Reducing Spice Mix

- 2 tablespoons whole coriander seeds
- 2 tablespoons turmeric powder
- 1 tablespoon whole cumin seeds
- 1 tablespoon ginger powder
- 1 tablespoon cinnamon powder
- 1 teaspoon clove powder
- 1 teaspoon ground black pepper

Note: You can also play with adding cayenne, chili powder, or paprika for a spicier blend.

Preparation instructions for spice mixes:

In a dry skillet, toast the whole seeds (except cardamom) until aromatic. Transfer seeds to a spice grinder and add cardamom seeds; process to a fine powder. Mix with powdered spices in a bowl and store in a glass container.

• • Essential Ideas • •

- A living, loved kitchen produces prana-filled food. When you love being in your kitchen, your food will hold more of that positive emotion. That positive prana will in turn, infuse your body and mind with vitality.
- There is nothing sexier than a body that has been infused with lovingly prepared foods, full of medicinal spices. Spices are truly sexy.
- Every meal is an opportunity to give your body medicine. Spices are Nature's secret agent for combatting and preventing disease and imbalances.

- Setting up a living kitchen with some basic kitchen tools and Ayurveda-inspired items for your pantry will make it easier to make healthy meals for yourself and your family.

Putting Ayurveda to Work

- Review the spices/herbs list in this chapter and choose 2–3 that are good for your current imbalance or constitution or time of year. Add them to your shopping list.
- Stock your kitchen with matching storage containers. I love using Mason jars. You can create beautiful labels for your dry goods, teas, spices, and churnas.
- Make a spice blend!

Part III

Happy

*A*yurveda teaches us that happiness is easy when we possess *svastha*, a word meaning "to be established in the soul." And reaching this state isn't some mountaintop experience where you attain enlightenment and return back home, suddenly and forevermore "established in your soul." This state of consciousness emerges slowly as a result of moment-by-moment routines and habits we choose over a lifetime.

This section will offer some of Ayurveda's best golden nuggets for your journey toward happiness. Through cultivating steady, Nature-loving routines in the nitty-gritty of modern daily life, we become more balanced. Healing self-care routines, exercise, and meditation are key players in the daily practices that will turn you into a happy, glowing goddess. When we connect with these daily routines that empower balance, it becomes so much easier to rest in our soul. And when we rest in our soul, our purpose in life becomes clear, our mind becomes calmer, and our heart feels nourished. These elements are fertile soil in which happiness blossoms. And there is nothing more beautiful, nothing sexier, than a woman who is happy.

My Own Evolution toward Happy

All my life, I've wanted to be happy. And if you have a beating heart, somewhere deep down inside you, you want the same thing. We all do. If we dig deep enough, we find that everything we do in life springs from a longing to be happy.

When I was a child I had immense amount of passion, creativity, and a natural sense of awe and curiosity about the world around me and beyond. But somewhere around late high school and college, I began to fall into certain habits that slowly degraded this natural, childlike vivacity. Like many of you reading this book, college was a time when I started staying out late, drinking booze, and eating too much junk food (hello, "freshman 15"). I went to college in Spain and spent much of those four wondrous years in sangria-soaked bars, smoking cigarettes, eating *jamon*, making out with boys named Alvaro, and staying out till sunrise. And while I look back with nostalgia upon those vino-stained years, I do see that they were unhealthy—and I was really, *really* unhappy.

By the time I started my job in the technology world, I had become firmly entrenched in habits that squelched my joy. And as I looked around at the people I worked with, I saw that they too relied on many different types of unhealthy crutches to get through the day. We all needed espresso to wake up from those long Spanish nights. And then we needed alcohol to calm down at the end of a long day sitting in front of a computer.

What happened? Where was the endless amount of creativity and vivacity so easily accessed when we were younger? How was it possible to be living a fairy-tale life and yet be so miserable? I had a killer job, lived in an apartment on the beach in the south of Spain, and worked with super-smart people, yet I felt like something was off. I wanted my "happy" back.

As I write these words, I am reminded of how much of that child-like joy has returned to me through the practices of Ayurveda and yoga. The more I practice Ayurveda the more a natural state of happiness shines through my body and mind. The more I give myself to the routines I will share with you in this section, the less I really strive for the external promises of a world that has forgotten Spirit. The more I give of myself through sharing these ancient rituals of a woman's well-being, the more Nature gives back to me. Her currency? Energy, vitality, and a type of joy that radiates from within.

9

Glowing Goddess Routines

Regular, nature-inspired routines are the body's best medicine. When I say routine, you may think of a bored factory worker tediously repeating the same movements on the line, day after day. But far from being life-draining, Ayurveda's daily to-do list affirms life by embracing the idea that routine asks us to remember the sacred. What would your life look like if every repetitive act were done as a prayer to inner and outer Divinity? If we are able to taste even the tiniest drop of the beautiful mystery of life as we brush our teeth or chop vegetables, we come close to heavenly bliss right here on Earth.

Try doing the suggested routines in this chapter with a sense of the sacred, but do not feel guilty if you don't get them right every day. In fact, it's better to take a few of the suggestions and work with them until they become second nature, rather than trying to do everything at once, failing miserably, and sending yourself to guilty town.

Aligning with Daily Subtlety

It's easy to get excited about a new program. You feel supported and ready to make changes. The same thing happens when we go on a great retreat or a workshop with an inspiring teacher. We feel juiced up and ready to make the changes that will bring us closer to our goals in life. But what happens? Over time, the bright fire burns out and we lose the momentum. We fall into the old routine because it is familiar and comfortable. A daily routine will keep your efforts consistent. Ayurvedic texts call daily routine a *dinacharya*. I'm giving you my version of this routine, tailored to a modern lady's life. Print this

111

baby up. Post it in your bathroom or on your fridge until practicing it becomes second nature!

Starting the Day with Love for Yourself

Your daily routine begins the night before: Getting in bed by 10:00 or 10:30 PM (or a little later in the summer) will help you start the morning off right.

- **Wake up at sunrise.** If you are exhausted, sick, or elderly, please sleep as long as you like. Upon waking, do not get out of bed right away. Try to be aware of your body and feel grateful to be alive before your toes touch earth.
- **Drink warm lemon water.** This helps to wash the gastrointestinal (GI) tract, flushes the kidneys, and stimulate peristalsis. If your digestion is sluggish, add ½ teaspoon gingerroot powder.
- **Nature calls.** Going to the bathroom upon waking will help clear your digestive system. A healthy movement will have a soft brown log quality, little odor, and will be well formed (like a banana). Undigested food, foul odor, mucus, excessive dryness, or a pellet-like quality suggests digestive imbalance. Altering your diet and lifestyle and using herbs will help improve this. (More on getting the perfect poo on page 73.)
- **Gently scrape your tongue.** Buy a stainless steel tongue scraper. Scrape from back to front 5–8 times. The tongue is a mirror of your intestines. When there is a thick white coating on the tongue, it is indicative that ama (toxins) is present. Tongue scraping helps prevent diseases of the oral cavity, improves our ability to taste, gets rids of old food debris, and prevents bad odor in the mouth.
- **Wash your face, mouth, teeth, and eyes.** Splash your face with cool water. Wash the eyes with cool water or real-deal rose water. You can also buy an eye cup at most pharmacies for washing the eyes. Massage your gums with sesame oil. This improves

oral hygiene, prevents bad breath, increases circulation to gums, heals bleeding gums, and helps us maintain strong, healthy teeth.

- **Use a neti pot.** Add ½ teaspoon salt to warm water in the pot and drain through each nostril. Afterward, put 3–5 drops of warm sesame oil or ghee in the nostrils to lubricate the nose. This keeps the sinuses clean and improves vocal, visual, and mental clarity. Our nose is the door to the brain. Nose drops nourish our prana and enhance intelligence.
- **Abhyanga (self-massage)** is one of our greatest allies for total health. It nourishes and soothes the nervous systems, stimulates lymphatic flow, and aids in detoxification. It also improves circulation, increases vitality, nourishes the skin, and promotes body/ mind balance. See page 141 for full directions on self-massage. One of our greatest allies in moving toward balance, exercise boosts the immune system and is an excellent way to counteract depression. Exercise daily to half capacity. We want to get a little sweaty glow but not burn out before our day begins.
- **Bathe, using natural products.**
- **Begin your day with some form of breath-work and meditation.** See chapter 12 for how-to's. Start with 5 minutes and work up to at least 20 minutes daily. I sometimes do my meditation before exercise. This is also fine.
- **Eat breakfast.**

Lunch Routines

Try to make lunch your biggest meal of the day. Eat in a pleasant, calm place without distraction.

Take some time to bless the food prior to eating.

After eating, if you can, lie down on your left side for 5–20 minutes. This is ideal. Why? Because it helps the digestive organs do their work to assimilate the meal. If you are at work, even just leaning to the left side in your chair will be helpful.

Afternoon/Early Evening Routines

One afternoon routine that helps you deeply relax into your evening is the practice of yoga nidra—a yogi nap. See the resources section for a recording from Para Yoga's Rod Stryker. It's also nice to do this prior to dinner, just before sunset.

Eat lightly at night. Having your last meal before sundown, and at least 3 hours before bedtime, will ensure better sleep. If you don't feel hungry, drink one of my nighty-night tonics in the Kitchen Pharmacy appendix of this book.

Nighty-Night Routines

There is no excuse for us to not be sleeping. Women need sleep. Men need sleep. Everybody on the planet needs 7-8 hours of sleep on a regular basis. Just as we need to exercise, we also need to surrender into rest.

It is impossible to accomplish your goals if you are chronically sleep deprived. Plus, your mind and body use sleep as the washing machine for the subconscious mind. If we aren't slipping into deep dreamtime every night, much of our toxic, unprocessed emotions and experiences don't get drained away. As Dr. Robert Svoboda says, "Sleep is known as the wet nurse of society."[1] Raise your hand if you feel like you need to be wet-nursed.

Ayurveda offers an ideal way to transition from the activity of the day into the sacred chamber of sleep. Following these routines will make sleep come effortlessly, and will help keep you asleep through the night:

1. **Set the mood.** Depending on the season (in the winter it may be earlier), start turning off overhead lights after dinner. Avoid fluorescent lights always, but especially at night. Low lighting helps tell your body it is time to go to sleep. Lots of light confuses your circadian rhythms and messes with the natural hormones

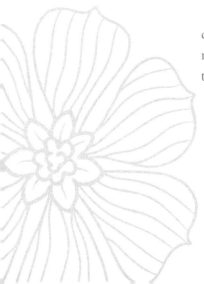

that pull you into the "sleepy feeling." One of the first questions I ask people who suffer from insomnia is, "Are your overhead lights still on at 8:00 and 9:00 PM?" Switch to low-level lighting or candles, or install dimmers on your overhead lights to set the mood for sleep.

2. **No more screen time.** Set an intention to turn off all screens (computers, cellphones, TVs) by 8:00 or 9:00 PM. Experts state that when we are exposed to artificial lighting (such as from computer and smartphone screens), the sleep-promoting hormone melatonin is suppressed, making us feel more alert and changing our circadian rhythms.[2]

3. **Be in bed by 10:00 PM.** Have you ever noticed that you get a second wind around 10:30 PM? That's because the metabolic energy your body normally uses for detoxing you while you sleep gets diverted to mental energy, and we get activated. Our body detoxifies and rejuvenates from 10:00 PM–2:00 AM. When we stay up late, we truly do miss out on beauty sleep. If you currently go to bed at midnight, use the 15-minute rule. Each night, try going to bed a mere 15 minutes earlier. Within a few weeks, you will be soundly sleeping at 10:00 PM.

4. **Take a warm bath.** Taking a scented warm bath can help reset the nervous system toward sleep. Use oils such as frankincense, myrrh, lavender, honeysuckle, chamomile, neroli, or pure rose for deep slumber.

5. **Avoid too much mental stimulation.** Don't watch evening news. It's toxic for your dreams. Similarly, avoid planning your future, having intense conversations, or any other activity that promotes mental movement before bed.

6. **Light a candle, read a sweet book that makes your heart melt, say some prayers, and turn in.**

7. **Unravel the day.** There is a powerful meditative practice for unraveling the day. It actually builds your power of assimilation and boosts memory. Once in bed and lying down, mentally go backward through your day in increments of 30 minutes. Try to

simply register what was happening to you during the day without judgment. Notice your feelings, relax, and let all events go. End with the point where you woke up in the morning. Gently drift into sleep.

Aligning with Seasonal Subtlety

Nature thrives in her cyclical routines. In fact, She is very predictable. And although Her Wild Highness can throw a tornado into the mix, She usually gives us clear indications of her changes if we open our eyes to her subtlety. The more we can align with these rhythms, the easier it is to maintain body/mind health. The word for seasonal routine in Sanskrit is *rutucharya*.

Rutucharya is not only related to the four seasons and the temperature outside. You may have noticed that life has its own seasonal flavor. You know, "to every thing (turn, turn, turn) there is a season." Yes, from life, death, heat, cold, night, day, orgasms, breakups, and firm breasts to crow's feet, the Ayurvedic sages noticed natural changes both in terms of how the cycles of the seasons relate to the earth's axis, and of how people cycle through their own life in a continuous experience of expansiveness and contraction.

As we begin to notice Nature's rhythms, we become more and more powerful. We tap into the Most Powerful One—Nature Herself. We also learn how to simultaneously work with the changes in our own bodies. We learn how to surrender to the inevitable beauty in the impermanence of everything. The good news? One of the Sanskrit roots inside the word for routine, rutucharya, is *turiya*, a word meaning "the imperishable love that rests, transcendent, beyond the routines." Change continually shows us its relationship to changelessness. And that is the goal, sisters: to honor the changing routine, so as to see what lies beyond it.

The ancient teachings encourages us to embrace mundane routines as a way of seeing even the most simple and repetitive aspects of life as sacred.

Seasonal Changes

As time passes, our state of mind as well as our physical body undergoes vast changes. Seasonal changes have a direct influence on all of earth's creatures, and change can be tough. Traditional societies understood this and created season-based rituals and celebrations to ease the shift. By getting together, sharing food, and honoring the changes, we experienced a kind of group catharsis that lifts individual consciousness, making it easier to weather the seasons.

Today, we have less and less of these critical rituals. We blow cold air through our vents in the heat of summer, and warm our bones with electric blankets in the winter. And while these technological advances definitely have their advantages, the downside of our useful man-made devices is that they disconnect us from the intimate and language-less relationship between the human body and the natural world. And this connection is crucial for our well-being. Sometimes we need to feel the drip of sweat pour between our breasts, smell the deep hot earth of July, and say, "Yes, this is summer, living in me and outside of me."

Okay, enough philosophy. Here is your Earth-Mama-Savvy guide to all things seasonal. Remember, this guide is general and subject to geography. If you happen to live in the tropics, or in the Arctic, you may also experience the subtle shifts in seasons and can adapt as appropriate.

Late Winter/Early Spring's Sweetness

In late winter and early spring, the Water element is predominant, although it is accompanied by the warming aspect of the sun (Fire element). When we are in balance in the springtime, we feel the inherent enthusiasm, rebirth, seed planting, cleansing, and creativity of the season. The cold darkness of winter is melted away by the first warm spring suns. Rivers get fatter, bees start to pollinate flowers, and human beings begin to feel the sensual pull of the season's strong creative desire. To all this bulging enthusiasm, a little spring rain must fall. Because of the watery warmth of the season, spring is notorious for bringing on allergies, colds, flu, mucus, stagnation, congestion, sluggishness, and even lascivious sexual impulses and overeating. These imbalances are especially true for early spring, when kapha is highest.

Routines for a Buoyant Inner Spring Fling

- Spend time outdoors.
- Plan marriages, new projects, and new purchases, as springtime is the season for new beginnings, rebirth, and renewal. Redecorate a room. Start a garden.
- Try waking shortly before or with the sunrise.
- Stay warm, particularly in the beginning of spring. You may feel tempted to bare it all out of the sheer joy of feeling the sultry sun on your wintry-white skin, but think twice. Spring brings a tendency for cool dampness to build up, particularly in the lungs.
- Exercise. Spring is the season where a more vigorous exercise routine makes the most sense. It is a time when the body naturally wants to shed excess winter blubber. Your lymphatic system will love a fluid yoga class, jumping rope, a bike ride, or a brisk walk.

Spring is the season extraordinaire for doing a dietary cleanse. I am not a fan of unguided, "do-it-yourself" cleanses. While a daylong cleanse is safe for most people, any longer cleanses should be done with the help of a reputable Ayurvedic practitioner. Why? Because while the cleanse may seem mellow, it is designed to "bring shit up"—literally and figuratively. I encourage you to meet with an Ayurvedic professional who can work with you to make sure you remain healthy and balanced during and after this life-changing undertaking.

Clean out your heart (and your garage). Spring is not just the time for cleansing the physical vessel. It is also a good time to let go of unhealthy habits, lovers, and for God's sake ladies, let's have a big old yard sale for all that junk in your basement. I love you, but hoarding is not hot.

Honor your desires. Spring is when we are intuitively most attuned to our deepest driving desires. This is especially true during late spring when the fire element builds. We may find ourselves with more hunger (sexually or in regard to food, as well as our drive and ambition in the world.) This is a good thing. It's almost as if the Big Mama were giving us some big birthing pushes, and if we can ride Her contractions, we can use the natural rhythm of spring to move forward in activity and accomplishment.

In general, diet should be seasonal and local. Eat from the kapha-reducing food list on page 66.

Summer's Heat

In the summer, the Fire element is predominant. When we are in balance in the summer, we can enjoy the season's inherent passion and fire. We can also quickly get too caught up in the solar energy and subsequently burn out. When I lived in Spain, I was always amazed watching Nordic tourists arrive at the sultry southern coasts. Like pagan sun worshippers, they could not be moved away from midday rays, all the while their skin turned a crispy langoustine red as they sipped their sangria (fire-juice anyone?). It's not a stretch to imagine that many a blonde babe found herself in the arms of a steamy Latin lover on those August nights. And it makes sense. We like feeling warm, golden, and satisfied. We just have to take care so we do not end up overheated, fire-engine red, and hungover.

Summer's imbalance can lead to increases in fiery conditions such as acne, rash, heatstroke, hives, or emotions of anger and intensity, as well as digestive upsets such as peptic ulcers, colitis, diarrhea, excess sweating, and boils.

Routines for Cooling Summer's Fire Princess

- Take your intense summer soul out for a moon bath. Pitta is reduced by gazing at the moon with a cool head and a loving heart. Swim in the moonlight for an assuredly pitta-reducing experience.
- Spray yourself with flower water. Buy a rose- or jasmine-water spritzer and use abundantly.

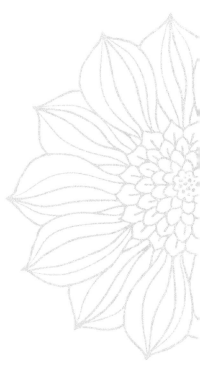

- Exercise in a way that won't spark the flame (especially if you already have a pitta body type). Regular exercise is important. Yoga and swimming are best during the hot season. Keep it slow and cool. Emphasize spinal twists and forward bends. This will help release excess Fire and toxins from the digestive system. Only exercise daily to half of your capacity in summer, just to the point where you get a little sweat glow going. I know this is hard for you intense pitta types, but your overall health will thank you in the long run.

- Cover your sumptuous skin in coconut oil. First of all, it makes you feel like you are on a cheaper version of a tropical vacation. Secondly, coconut oil is cooling and has natural detoxification and nourishment properties. Gentle daily self-massage with coconut oil will not only slow your roll and cool your intensity, it will also promote healthy aging, calm the nervous system, and reduce dehydration. See page 141 for self-massage how-to's. Emphasize seasonal foods that are cool, dry, and heavy. Emphasize sweet, bitter, and astringent tastes. Eat from the pitta-reducing food list on page 63.

- Drink cool (not iced) water with mint, cucumber, or lime.

- Avoid intensity and conflict in the already-heated July and August months. It's best not to make decisions about a divorce in the heat of the summer. Remember, heat and passion peak at midday when the sun is highest, as well as from 10:00 PM–2:00 AM. Romance is wonderful in the summer. But too much sex can overheat us. Tell your partner you want more cuddling.

- Rose, lavender, jasmine, lotus, sandalwood, and hibiscus are cooling fragrances that feed your Mama Spirit and the feminine heart. You can use them as essential oils, powders, teas, or fresh flowers.

- Fashion is your friend. Wear cooling colors. White, blue, or light-green, loose-fitting clothing of cotton or silk is great for mitigating summer's heat.

- Sleep on the right side to cool the nervous system.

The Fall/Early Winter Season

In fall, the Air element is dominant. It is the vata tim
a windy autumn day. The air is dry, cool, and movir
increase during the fall and winter seasons in na
our individual nature as well.

Fall and early winter remind us of impern
season is windy, emptying, rough, and dry. If
feel our mind and body undergoing a shift toward a n.
Like a turtle drawing its head into a protective shell, winter .
for intuition, stillness, and dying off. When out of balance in winter, we
can tend toward the more vata-genic conditions of constipation, fear,
cracking joints, arthritic pain, dry skin, anxiety, insomnia, and seasonal
sadness (due to the lack of sunlight). How you care for yourself during
the fall season will determine your body's ability to maintain health
through winter. Winter is the time to keep warm, oiled-up, nourished,
and protected.

Routines for Warming Fall/Early Winter's Inner Hearth

- Stoke your digestive fire (agni). See page 73 for how-to's.
- Sip warm ginger tea throughout the day.
- Give yourself an oil massage every morning. This will benefit
  your skin and help ground the Air energy that causes anxiety or
  sleeplessness or both. Sesame oil is an excellent winter oil, as it
  is both nourishing and warming. Mahanarayan oil, another great
  warming oil, is particularly good for aching joints and pain.
- Take a warming bath with ginger powder to stimulate your body.
- Go to bed between 9:00 and 10:00 PM. Getting sufficient rest
  is the number-one remedy for increasing the immune power
  of the body. Only in winter can we really let ourselves sleep as
  much as needed. In fact, our not-so-distant ancestors enjoyed
  an amazing amount of sleep during the colder months. Because
  there was no heat and electricity, it was not uncommon to sleep
  14–15 hours a night.

- Layer up. It may seem like common sense, but keep yourself warm.
- Avoid wearing too much black or dark blue during winter. We all love fashionable, slimming black, but keep in mind that this color absorbs all light. Too much black leaves us with a feeling of vastness and emptiness—a feeling already heightened during winter.
- Avoid all raw and cold foods such as salad, ice water, and smoothies in winter. Come on, mama, you know that your great-grandma was not eating salad in the wintertime, and there was good reason for that.
- Be okay with lying low. With the holidays at hand, we tend to spin out of balance in winter more than any other season. What were once local ritual traditions where families would meet to share in the warmth of home, hearth, and nurturing stews has now turned into the season of consumer-crazy spending, over-booked party calendars, plane flights, and family dramas. Try creating more gentle holiday traditions. Keep it as local as possible. Stay inside. Light a fire.
- Before bed, enjoy a mild sedative such as the hot spiced medicinal milk (see recipes section). Add ½ teaspoon of ghee for even more vata-soothing and ojas (immunity) boosting properties.
- Avoid loud music, excessive exercising, too much sex, traveling, leftovers, cleansing, fasting, and over-talking.
- Exercise can be a little more active and warming in the cold of winter. This is a good time to practice warmer forms of yoga, if you are so inclined. Emphasizing backbends and laterals will keep your spirits awake and alive in what can be a dark time of year.

Beloved Boobies

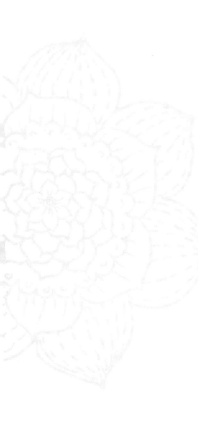

The breasts hold a prominent role in our female collective psyche, both as sexual pleasure site and a sacred archetype of mothering. How is it, then, that we spend more time nourishing our teeth than our breasts? Ayurveda encourages us to develop a loving relationship and routine around the feminine parts of our bodies. Such a routine can help balance hormones, prevent disease, and reconnect you to your sexuality and femininity.

I strongly recommend massaging the breasts in castor or sesame oil to stimulate circulation, promote lymphatic flow, and reduce any buildup of ama in the breast tissue.[3] I keep a bottle of castor oil in the shower and give my breasts a nice massage daily. Lady's mantle, fenugreek, calendula, and bladder wrack are also wonderful herbs to be infused into the oils for breast protection. I recommend Banyan Botanical's Breast Balm or Lady Nada's Breast Oil from Rupam's Apothecary (see resources section). I also recommend the book *Balance Your Hormones, Balance Your Life* by Dr. Claudia Welch for a more in-depth look at breast cancer prevention and research.

Use about a teaspoon of your oil on each breast, depending on the size. Massage in an upward circular motion from the outer lower quadrant of the breast, across the bottom of the breast, toward your heart, around, up, and back outward toward the underarm. Pay particular attention to the area under the armpits. Massaging the breasts in this way cleanses the tissue of ama, breaks up cysts and stagnation, and encourages lymph movement. It also cultivates body love and self-awareness around any changes in your breast tissue. When you massage your breasts, it sends a subconscious message to your female essence. Your inner goddess whispers, "Your breasts are perfect, whether you look like Twiggy or Marilyn Monroe."

Other Beautiful Breast Routines

- Ditch the underwire bras. Wires enslave the boobies and cut off the flow of prana, constricting blood and lymph flow and creating an environment for disease. If you have larger breasts and this simply isn't an option, make sure to never sleep in underwire bras and give your breasts plenty of massage and breathing time.[4]
- Throw out any antiperspirants lurking in your bathroom cabinets. Antiperspirants clog the critical lymph area around the armpits.

This keeps the area from detoxifying, sending toxins back toward breast tissue. Use all-natural, aluminum-free deodorants.

- For thousands of years, Ayurveda-inspired women have been using this fenugreek mix for perky, firm breasts: Place ¼ cup fenugreek powder into a bowl (more if your breasts are large). Add enough water to make a paste and mix well. Massage onto breasts. Leave for 5-15 minutes and then rinse off.
- Avoid caffeine. During cultivation, coffee beans are often heavily sprayed with estrogenic chemicals and pesticides that can disrupt breast health.

Taking Care of the Eyes

Ayurveda is unique in its approach to taking care of one of our most important sense organs. Rather than simply treating the eye itself, Ayurveda believes that the images we take in on the visual plane can affect the health of our eyes. This is why it is important to see beautiful things on a daily basis—a bronze sunset, a bird's yellow breast, steam coming off the surface of a hot spring. What is more, the skin around our eyes is also prone to imbalance, as it is one of the most delicate tissues of the body. Vata imbalances in eyes lead to early eye-area-wrinkling (crow's feet), dryness, and nervous eye tics. Pitta imbalances relate to anything hot, itchy, or red around the eyes. Kapha imbalances bring about eye mucus, swelling, unclear vision, and general puffiness in the eye area.

Recipes for Happy Eyes

Do *trataka*. A simple and powerful practice for eye health, this ancient technique not only burns the impurities of the eyes, but also awakens intuition and inner vision. Try doing trataka at night, as it will calm the mind before bed. This is also an excellent practice for people who spend a lot of time staring at screens. Stop and practice trataka for a few minutes before returning to your work. Here are the steps:

1. Light a candle and put in on the floor, a small low meditation table, or a stack of books in front of you at about arm's length. The goal is to have the candle as close to eye height as possible. Sit in a comfortable position with your spine straight.

2. Begin with your eyes closed, allowing your awareness to relax and follow the movement of some deep breaths.

3. When you feel a deeper stillness in the mind/body, allow your eyes to open and let your gaze rest at the tip of the candle's wick. Keep your eyes open and focused. Try not to blink or move the eyes.

4. Hold this gaze for as long as possible. After a few minutes, your eyes will begin to water. The healing process has begun. Keep the gaze for a minute more, allowing the eyes to water.

5. After a minute or so, or when your eyes tire, close them and rest. Work up to doing 2–4 rounds of this practice.

Here are some other helpful daily routines you can follow to maintain happy eyes:

- Ditch the chemicals. Mascara, eyeliner, eye shadow, and chemical makeup removers are really hard on the eyes. Make sure to only use mineral-based makeup. To remove makeup, use a natural organic cream or sunflower oil.

- Wash your eyes in the morning with an eyecup and rinse, which can be purchased at any pharmacy. Use cool water or organic rose water in the eye cup.

- Give your eyes a ghee bath. As we age, our eyes become more and more strained. Computers screens speed up the aging process of the eyes. Giving your eyes a ghee-soak helps to reduce eye strain and strengthen the vision. Soak 4 cotton balls in some melted ghee until fully saturated. Place 2 over each of your closed eyes, lie back and relax for at least 15 minutes, allowing the ghee to slowly seep into the eyes. Cucumbers are a natural astringent, meaning that they help pull excess water and puffiness from the tissues. They also have a hydrating effect on the skin, meaning that they can pull out the old and bring in new, clean water. Cucumbers are also cooling for the sensitive skin of the eyes, and help reduce excessive mental heat. Crush a small piece of peeled cucumber and place the pulp around the eyes. You can also juice a cucumber, soak a few cotton balls in the liquid and place them on your closed eyes for 15–20 minutes.

Hair Care:
Is Your Shampoo Making You Fat?

Okay, so maybe there's not a direct connection between shampoo and weight, but I knew it would get your attention—and hopefully get you thinking. Studies are now showing that there is a possible relationship between the products we use every day, the chemicals inside them, the disruption of our hormone balance in the human body, and the destruction of the fish in the sea. And it's pretty common knowledge that big companies pump products full of gnarly chemicals.

Avoid any product like the plague if it contains:[5]

- **Urea:** A preservative that releases formaldehyde, a known carcinogen
- **Diethanolamine (DEA) and triethanolamine (TEA):** Gnarly carcinogenic chemicals connected to multiple forms of cancer
- **Formaldehyde:** A known carcinogen and allergen
- **Parabens:** Super-common preservatives that have been linked to breast cancer
- **Phthalates:** Known to wreak havoc on major organ tissues, including the liver, kidneys, lungs, and reproductive organs, phthalates have also been connected to breast cancer, birth defects, and reduced sperm counts.
- **Mineral oil:** A petroleum by-product that suffocates skin's natural ability to breathe. It is full of carcinogens linked to breast cancer.

- **Propylene glycol and polyethylene glycol (PEG):** Basically these are cancer-causing antifreezes
- **Sodium lauryl (laureth) sulfate:** Allergy-boosting carcinogen that mimics the activity of estrogen. This has been linked to increased PMS, infertility, and breast cancer.
- **Synthetic fragrances:** Some of the worst allergens on the planet
- **Synthetic colors:** Carcinogenic skin irritants

These chemicals get into our bodies and bloodstreams and create an estrogenic effect that mimics natural estrogen—only it's not. Then, our bodies are confused because of excess fake estrogen, causing us to produce excess emotion and too much of some types of tissues that are harmful (aka excess fat, excess emotion, and excess bad tissue that can turn into tumors).

The bottom line is that the synthetic aromas we put into products are gross and could be making us feel fat, sick, and anxious. So, what's that got to do with fish? Well, remember, your body contains all of the elements and energies present in nature. Your beautiful body is a microcosm of Mother Nature. When you have excess chemical fake estrogens in the river of your blood, Big Mama has excess chemicals in Her own rivers. Just like those chemicals create imbalances in our cells and tissues, the runoff of the shampoo in your drain creates phytoestrogenic waters in our oceans and rivers that blast fish with heaping helpings of our chemical consumerism. And scientists inform us that many fish and other animal populations are seeing a "feminization" of the species, as high levels of endocrine-disrupting chemicals begin to neuter males.[6] This is serious stuff. And if you are anything like me, the last thing we want is a world full of neutered males!

Here are some DIY shampoos. If you don't have time to make them yourself, there are some excellent, Earth-Mama-Lovin' products in the resources section.

Absolute Beauty's Dry Shampoo[7]: Mix equal parts cornmeal, almond meal, and orris root. Massage into dry scalp and brush out, or shake off, excess.

Weekly Hair Mask: Mix 1 teaspoon each of *amalaki*, neem, and licorice powder with 8 teaspoons rose water or plain water. Apply the paste to your scalp and hair. Leave for one hour and rinse thoroughly.

Heavenly Hair Oils

Oiling the hair is the single best way to keep it healthy. The head is composed of multiple stress-relieving energy points. Oiling the head helps energize the mind, relieve stress, reduce scalp dryness and dandruff and strengthens hair roots. Oiling also helps pull out any excess heat accumulated in the head and mind. Simply oiling your hair and head can help boost your ojas, as it relaxes us, helps us sleep, and can even improve memory. I recommend doing a hair-oiling ritual once a week. Make sure to stay warm while oiling your head, as this process is cooling for the body. Do not oil your scalp when you are cold or sick. Remember, oiling the hair can be something of a meditation. Spend about 20 minutes relaxing or meditating with your head oiled.

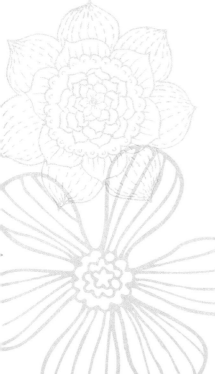

- **Simple Coconut Hair Oil:** Warm a little pure organic coconut oil and gently massage 3–5 tablespoons (depending on your hair's length and thickness) into the scalp. Then, comb the oil through the hair to the ends. Apply a towel that does not mind a little oil, or wear a plastic shower cap. Leave the coconut oil on your hair for at least 20 minutes (or overnight) before washing it out.
- **Decadent Coconut Hair Oil:** For a richer experience, bring 1 cup of coconut oil to about 100°F in a small pan on your stovetop. Remove from heat and add 6 tablespoons of pure rose water and 1 cup fresh flower petals (I recommend rose, jasmine, lavender, marigold, or hibiscus). Return the mixture to a boil and cook for 3 minutes. Let the flower petals steep in the oil for at least 24 hours, strain with a fine mesh strainer, and store in a glass bottle with a lid. Use in the same manner as the Simple Coconut Hair Oil.

Taking Care of Your Nose

Nasya is an ancient practice of placing medicated herbs and decoctions into the nose. Ayurveda sees the nose as the closest entrance to the brain and a key entry point into higher consciousness. For this reason, nasal treatments were highly revered as sacred practice for clearing out the channels of prana to the brain. This technique offers a multitude of health benefits for the modern woman—it can be used to treat nasal dryness; neck, head, and shoulder tightness; headaches; and hoarseness in the voice, and it moistens the sinuses. Doing this quirky practice is even said to nourish the energy that boosts our intelligence, reduces anxiety and insomnia, improves our vision, and enhances our voices. Science supports this ancient practice. One recent study found that nasya offered a marked relief in 70 percent of patients suffering with chronic sinusitis.[8]

How to Do a Nasya

- Make sure to do this practice on an empty stomach. Eating directly after this practice is also not recommended. Wait at least 30 minutes.
- Warm a little sesame oil or ghee. Banyan Botanicals has an amazing herb-infused Nasya Oil that you can buy online.
- Lean your head back and place 4 or 5 drops of the warm oil into each nostril.
- When you feel the oil beginning to drain into the throat, return the head to neutral and wipe any excess oil off the nose.
- Do this practice in the morning and evening for best results.
- Do not use it if you are pregnant or menstruating.

The Notorious Neti Pot

Despite its somewhat intimidating phallic appearance, the neti pot is one of ancient Ayurveda's greatest gifts to modern-day humans, and benefits all three doshas. With all the exhaust fumes and chemical toxicants we

How to Use a Neti Pot

Recent evidence has shown that modern water sources may not be clean enough for use in the neti pot. Make sure to use only distilled water, or boil your water before using so as to prevent getting any contamination in the sensitive tissues of the nose, ears, and brain.

To use a neti pot: Fill the pot with warm water, adding ½ teaspoon of sea salt. Place the spout at the edge of one of the nostrils and tilt the head to the side and slightly forward, so that the water moves through the nostril and out the other side. It may feel like you are drowning at first, but over time you will get used to it. Just make sure to breathe through your mouth, and not your nose. Do one pot per nostril.

are exposed to on a daily basis, this little ceramic pot may be our greatest hope for cleaning out the gunk we hold in those two little nasal openings. Allergy sufferers will also get tremendous relief by making nasal care with a neti pot part of the daily routine. It can also help clear your nasal passage for deeper breathing in asana and pranayama. Mystically speaking, it opens the channels of the third eye, promoting deeper meditation.

Mouth Care

Ayurveda has seen the link between oral health and overall immunity for thousands of years. Our mouths are a veritable breeding ground for bacteria and other harmful critters. Without proper daily mouth care, toxins can build up in our mouth and lead to other more serious health issues. Our immune system is constantly working to keep these toxins at bay. If we don't help our bodies by cleansing the mouth, these organisms can take over and lead to chronic inflammation. Studies show that ancient techniques of mouth care can help prevent many diseases today. Taking care of your mouth the Ayurveda way will help reduce cavities, plaque, and infections in your mouth. It can also help strengthen gum tissue and reduce the buildup of bacteria and fungus in the mouth.[9] This section will teach you how to keep your mouth happy and healthy with these Ayurvedic routines.

- First thing in the morning, before you even take your first sip of water or coffee, go to the bathroom and scrape your tongue from back to front with a stainless steel tongue scraper. This pulls off bacteria, old food, fungus, and other toxins, where they tend to accumulate as we sleep. It also pulls the bacteria-rich compounds off the back of the tongue. These are the gnarliest critters, and account for most cases of really bad breath.
- Always use a soft toothbrush. If your bristles are bristling-out, then it's time to buy a new one.

- Use a natural toothpaste such as Ayurdent, Auromère, Thera-Neem Organix, Vicco, or any brand that contains bitter neem or other cleansing herbals. Have you ever noticed how most toothpastes on the market are sweet? Ayurveda teaches us that it is the astringent (not sweet!) taste that strengthens the gums, and the bitter taste that kills viruses, bacteria, and fungus.
- Massage the gums with a little sesame oil. You can add a drop of clove, tea tree, or eucalyptus essential oils. This helps prevent bleeding gums and other forms of periodontal disease.
- Gargle with salt water.

Oil Pulling

Oil pulling involves holding or swishing pure unprocessed sesame or coconut oil in the mouth for around 15–20 minutes. Oil pulling is actually a fairly modern Ayurvedic practice for detoxing the teeth, gums, tongue, and throat as the pure oils act to "pull" out disease-causing critters. Scientific research shows that lipids in the oil pull out bacteria and fungus, preventing them from adhering to the walls of our mouth and gums.[10] It can also significantly reduce gingivitis, bacteria counts, and dental cavities.[11] And it's not just your mouth that reaps the benefits, but your whole body.

Amazingly, doing a cold-pressed natural oil mouthwash can actually boost cellular restructuring in your entire body. It increases the smooth functioning of the lymphatic and organ systems. By ridding the body of these toxins orally, oil pulling may help improve everything from migraine headaches, eczema, and hormonal imbalances, to more serious conditions such as arthritis and heart disease. Other reported benefits to oil pulling include increasing the strength of teeth and gums, preventing or treating cavities, gingivitis, tooth decay, bad breath, bleeding gums, dry mouth, and TMJ or jaw pain.[12] And if 20 minutes seems like an eternity, swish while you do something else, like laundry or making breakfast.

• • Essential Ideas • •

- Routine asks us to remember the sacred in day-to-day tasks.
- Daily and seasonal routines help us connect with the rhythms of nature. Ultimately, these routines are the best tools for boosting our total health and radiance.
- Try to do regular mouth care daily. If you can get in a few sessions of oil pulling and the neti pot as well, you are well on your way to Ayurvedic body-care happiness.
- Keep a bottle of castor oil in your shower to remind you to massage your breasts!

Putting Ayurveda to Work

To start, pick three things from the morning and night routines to introduce into your day.

Get out your journal and answer the following: What are some of the challenges you may have in implementing a new routine? How can you work with those challenges? For example, if you are having a hard time incorporating three elements of the morning routine because of a lack of time, can you go to bed 20–30 minutes early tonight and wake up earlier tomorrow?

Boost Radiance and Slow Aging

Every woman I know wants to be and feel beautiful. From an Ayurvedic standpoint, this makes perfect sense; Nature is beautiful, so it should come as no surprise that we would also desire to be as beautiful and radiant as possible. This longing represents a renewed communion with the deepest part of ourselves and the underlying reality of the cosmos.

Every woman I know is also at least a little annoyed about the warped, media-pushed mono-version of beauty we are fed on a daily basis. Billions of women see images that they will never look like. We see them in the line at the grocery store. We drive by them on billboards. They pop up on our computer screens as we innocently check our email. Mass advertising feeds us a daily diet of manufactured beauty that keeps us feeling bad about ourselves while simultaneously buying the products that we hope will finally "fix us."

The Ayurvedic view of beauty is different from the supermarket checkout lane version. The ancients saw that the more we could enliven our own robust nature through Ayurvedic lifestyle practices, the more we could become the embodiment of illuminating natural beauty. This beauty says, "I am healthy and connected to life." A woman holds an unmistakable radiance when she is connected to Nature and Her plants. This radiance, when combined with an authenticity of spirit, turns all women into real-beauty bombshells.

Whether or not we feel radiant and thriving (and hopefully even beautiful) is directly tied to how we *feel* in our body. And while previous chapters of the book taught us how to reconnect to the body and its beauty from the inside out, this chapter will emphasize an outside-in approach mainly related to the most important organ of our natural outer beauty—the skin. Ayurveda understands the importance of the skin. The skin is connected to our feelings of worthiness. The skin and other sense organs are gateways between the soul and the outside world. When we feel touched by life, our skin glows from the inside out. When we put natural, plant-based medicines on our skin and sense organs, these parts of us feel loved, and they start to glow.

With time and age, things tend to dry up. To slow this natural aging process and keep us feeling the glow of youth for longer periods of time, Ayurveda teaches us how to keep things as juicy as possible. Imagine your body as a series of channels full of a golden sap that is directly responsible for how juicy, wet, satisfied, and content you feel at any given time. Ayurveda calls this sap *rasa*, a Sanskrit word meaning "taste." Another meaning of the word is "contentment." Imagine it like a psychophysical honey charged with your life force. The word for rejuvenation in Ayurvedic therapy is *rasayana*, or as Ayurvedic expert Dr. Robert Svaboda translates it, "the path of juice." This chapter will teach you how to keep your skin as juicy as possible, the all-natural way.

Practical Beauty for Your Dosha

We can now apply all of our understanding of vata, pitta, and kapha to our skin care. Read these fresh-face tips for daily face beauty for all doshic types. Then, determine your skin dosha and have fun mixing up some all-natural face products in your kitchen.

Daily Tips for a Fresh, All-Natural Face

- Golden Rule of Skin: If you wouldn't eat it, you shouldn't put it on your body.
- Trade in your commercial makeup remover for sesame oil (dry skin) or sunflower oil (oily or sensitive skin). Never remove makeup with tissues or toilet paper. Use an all-natural sponge or soft cotton ball.

- Cleanse and oil your skin regularly. Try applying a doshic-appropriate face mask at least once a week for deeper cleansing and nourishing.
- Massage oils into your wet skin with gentle upward and outward strokes.
- Avoid stretching, scrubbing, or other abusive skin treatment. Treat your skin like a baby's, and it will look like a baby's.
- Avoid excess sun, wind, cold, and heat. If you are going to the beach or the pool, coat your skin and hair in a protective layer of coconut oil. You will still need sunscreen to prevent burning. Put sunscreen on first and let it dry before applying the coconut oil.
- Don't EVER let masks dry on your face. Keep them wet with a rose or lavender spray.
- Don't put anything on your face before bed. Heavy night creams clog the skin.
- Avoid chemical- and alcohol-based products.
- Avoid super hot or super cold water on your face.

What's My Skin Dosha?

In general, you have vata-type skin if:

- your skin tends toward early wrinkling and dryness
- you have combination skin (dry and oily)
- you have a thin bone structure, fine pores, and dark, scanty, or frizzy hair
- you tend toward nervous restless emotion, worry, movement, and creativity
- when out of balance, your skin tends toward excess dryness, wrinkles on forehead, dry eczema, psoriasis, and discoloration, as well as brittle nails and cracked lips
- when out of balance, your digestion tends toward constipation and gas

In general, you have pitta-type skin if:

- your skin tends toward inflammation and sensitivity
- you have a medium frame and lustrous skin, with oily T-zone and dry cheeks
- you have soft, moderately thick hair with light or reddish tones
- you are ambitious, a natural leader, intense, critical, and tend toward anger or irritation
- when out of balance, your skin tends toward excess whiteheads, rashes, acne rosacea, broken capillaries, or burning eczema
- when out of balance, your digestion tends toward loose stools

In general, you have kapha-type skin if:

- your skin is on the thick or clammy side
- you have a large frame and are prone to gaining weight
- you have soft skin with large pores
- you have thick, wavy, lustrous hair
- when out of balance, your skin tends toward excess oiliness, cystic acne, lack of tone, flabbiness, puffiness, excess sweat, and swollen eczema
- when out of balance, your digestion tends to be sluggish or contain mucus

Vata Face Nutrition

For cleansing vata-prone skin:

Mix ½ cup almond meal with ½ cup dry organic milk. For added nutrition, add 4 teaspoons brahmi powder. Mix and store in a glass, airtight container. Then, make a paste with a little water and 2 teaspoons of the mixture. Apply to face and gently massage into skin for one minute. Rinse with warm water. Use in the morning and evening.

For nourishing vata-prone skin:

Add 1 tablespoon of organic heavy whipping cream and 10 drops of rose, neroli, or jasmine essential oil to the above cleansing mixture. Massage into skin for about one minute and leave for a few minutes to allow the medicine to penetrate the skin. Use as needed. Keeps refrigerated for a few weeks.

For deep hydration of vata-prone skin:
Massage vata skin in small upward and outward gentle circles with pure organic, cold-pressed sesame oil (not toasted). Leave the oil on skin for at least 20 minutes. Rinse if needed. Do this daily.

Vata weekly mask:
Mash an avocado. Add 10 drops neroli or lemon essential oil. Slather on face. Lie down and do some deep belly breaths for 20 minutes. Rinse.

Pitta Face Nutrition

For cleansing pitta-prone skin:
Mix ½ cup almond meal with ½ cup dry organic milk. For added nutrition, add 3 teaspoons ground orange peel, 2 teaspoons ground sandalwood, and 1 teaspoon neem powder. Mix and store in an airtight glass container. Then, make a paste with a little water (or pure rosewater) and 2 teaspoons of the mixture. Apply to face and gently massage into skin for 1 minute. Rinse with cool water. Use in the morning and evening.

For nourishing pitta-prone skin:
Crush 3 tablespoons of organic cucumber and apply to face. Leave on for 20 minutes.

For deep hydration of pitta-prone skin:
Massage pitta skin with almond oil and leave oil on skin for at least 20 minutes. Rinse if needed. Do this daily.

Pitta weekly mask:
Mash a banana. Add 10 drops rose, sandalwood, or ylang-ylang essential oil. Slather on face. Lie down and do some deep belly breaths for 20 minutes. Rinse.

Kapha Face Nutrition

For cleansing kapha-prone skin:
Mix ½ cup barley meal with 2 teaspoons ground orange peel, 2 teaspoons ground fenugreek, and 2 teaspoons ground lemon peel. Mix and store in a glass, airtight container. Then, make a paste with a little water and 2 teaspoons of the mixture. Apply to face daily and gently massage into skin for 1 minute. Rinse with warm water. Use in the morning and evening.

For nourishing kapha-prone skin:
For added nutrition, add 2 teaspoons neem powder to the above cleansing mix. Add a little sunflower oil and 5–10 drops of lavender oil (enough to make a paste). Massage into skin for 1 minute and leave on for at least 10 minutes. Rinse with warm water.

For deep hydration of kapha-prone skin:
Kapha-prone skin rarely needs strong moisturizing. Try the kapha mask for deeper nourishment.

Kapha weekly mask:
Mash several large strawberries or papaya (this is particularly good for overly-oily skin of any type). Add 5 drops lavender essential oil and 5 drops clary sage oil. Slather on face. Lie down and do some deep belly breaths for 20 minutes. Rinse.

Rasa—The Sap of Life

As we said before, when we age we begin to lose some of the natural juiciness of youth. The body shrinks, the joints dry, and the mind loses sharpness and acuity as we move into the vata stage of life. But Ayurveda says this process can be dramatically slowed down, keeping us young and vital for longer periods of time. To counteract this aging, we use the "path of juice" to re-grease the machine with herb-infused oils. As *Caraka Samhita* (Vol. 1, V: 88–89) says:

The body of one who uses oil massage regularly does not become affected much even if subjected to accidental injuries or strenuous work. By using oil massage daily, a person is endowed with pleasant touch, trimmed body parts and becomes strong, charming, and least affected by old age.

The word for oil in Sanskrit is *sneha*. Another translation of the same word is "love" or "affection." You see, the essence of a plant is its oil, just as the essence of who we are is love. If we keep extracting something down to its purest essence, what remains is love. When we massage our body with oil, we are literally coating it with a layer of our affection, as well as a healing touch. This love is known as abhyanga, a simple form of self-massage.

Despite the ancient Caraka's beautiful promise of trimmed, strong, charming bodies, our beauty culture du jour has sold us the message, "Oily is gross." Anything unctuous or juicy is to be promptly astringed and exfoliated away, leaving no sign that underneath our expensive designer beauty products, we may be juice-producing, oil-secreting women. Ladies of the land, may we let this idea die, and may our new mantra be, "Oily is beautiful." Repeat: "Oily is beautiful." In fact, oil is what keeps the skin young, taut, and supple.

The truth is that the simple practice of oiling our physical machine is, quite possibly, the best thing we can do for the body and the nervous system on a daily basis. In fact, there is a phrase in traditional Indian healthcare that says, "Either pay the oil man today, or you will be paying the doctor tomorrow." And as our skin is the largest organ of the body (in fact, it weighs anywhere from 6 to 10 pounds), we may do well in caring for this large, biologically active organ.

There are significant benefits of doing self-massage with Ayurvedic oils

- Self-massage cleanses and soothes the body, including the nervous and endocrine systems.

- The skin is alive. It lives and breathes and heals itself. It removes waste from itself. By oiling our skin, we better its ability to breathe and thrive.
- You tap into touch. And touch is 10 times stronger than verbal or emotional contact. The skin is one of the primary seats of emotion, feelings, and desire.
- Self-massage stimulates important energy points and the cutaneous nerves throughout the skin that connect to every part of the body.
- When we self-massage, we release a cascade of feel-good, life-enriching growth factor hormones into our bloodstream. Research shows that massage can decrease cortisol, a stress hormone that can be degenerative when you have too much of it. Massage can also increase dopamine, oxytocin, ACTH (adreno corticotropic) and norepinephrine, all known mood boosters, that reduce anxiety and increase relaxation and pleasure.[1]
- It calms the nervous system, increases vitality, strengthens vision, prevents dehydration, nourishes the skin, remedies insomnia, and restores balance in the body and mind.
- The rubbing and stroking actions dislodge accumulated toxins and impurities from the body and move them into the digestive system.
- Massage stimulates our immune system.
- It acts as an effective medium for delivering plant medicine.
- It promotes free flow of prana.
- It lubricates and promotes flexibility of joints, muscles, and tissues.
- It rejuvenates the skin, promoting softness and luster.
- It promotes a radiant glow and healthy aging.

What Oil Should I Use?

The main thing we need to consider when working with oils is the condition of the skin. While you may have a predominance of the vata dosha in the heat of summer, it still may benefit you to use a cooling oil. I tell my students and clients to treat their skin, not their original dosha.

- Generally, vata skin is deeply healed and nourished by sesame oil.
- Generally, pitta skin is cooled and nourished by coconut and sunflower oil.
- Generally, kapha skin is enlivened by sunflower or calendula-infused oil.

Sometimes kapha skin is so moist that it doesn't require oil (especially in the springtime). In this case, dry brush the skin before showering.

How to Oil Your Bodacious Body

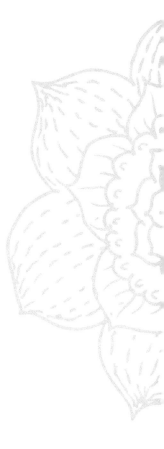

Start by warming your oil. We warm the oil because it cures it, allowing the oil to be more easily absorbed by the skin and tissues. There are a number of ways to cure the oil. The best way is to heat a small amount in a pan on low heat. You will know that the oil is done by throwing 1 drop of water on the oil. If it pops, it's cured. Let it cool a little before applying to your body. You can also heat the appropriate oil for your constitution in a double boiler. Or simply place the glass bottle directly in your bathroom sink, close the drain, and fill with the hottest water possible. Allow to sit for at least 10 minutes before applying to the body. If you are using essential oils, add them after you remove the oil from the heat, as we don't want to heat these delicate oils. Remove all clothing and jewelry. Sit on an old towel so as not to make a mess.

For the full bliss treatment, we would start at the top of the head and pour the oil directly onto the crown. If you are doing this before work and do not want an oily head for the rest of the day, you can skip this part and save it for a day when you do not need to be presentable. That said, Ayurvedic tradition places heavy emphasis on massaging the head and neck. Of the 107 energy points of the body (called *marmas*), 37 are located on the head and neck.

Continue gently massaging oil onto the face and the rest of the body. On the arms and legs, use back-and-forth strokes. On the joints, use circular strokes. On the belly, use circular strokes in a clockwise motion (if you are looking down at your belly) as this is the direction

Sianna Sherman's Ayurvedic Oiling Ritual

As I bathe myself in oil before showering, I say this prayer to the Goddess Durga out loud as I gently stroke smooth, warm oil over my body from my toes to my head.

My toes are the light of the sun.

My feet walk the sacred path of creation.

My legs are made from the power of water.

My hips are the light of the earth.

My waist is from the kingdom of heaven.

My breasts are made of moonlight.

My arms emerge from all that sustains.

My fingers are the children of creativity.

My teeth are from the Lord of creatures.

My nose is the blessing of the wealth of the senses.

My eyes are the light of fire.

My third eye is the light awakening.

My eyebrows are the sunrise and the sunset.

My ears are gifts from the wind.

My hair is the blessing of living life fully until my last breath.

My face is the light of pure awareness.

My whole body is the embodiment of Shakti's infinite power.

Then, in the shower as I'm washing, I chant the names, mantras, and songs of Durga and remember that She is me and I am Her.

(For Sianna Sherman's complete contribution to *Healthy Happy Sexy*, check out www.healthyhappysexylife.com.)

---

in which our long intestine moves, and will stimulate proper digestion.

Ideally, you want to spend 15-20 minutes massaging your body. If time is an issue, spend at least 5 minutes in total communion with your vehicle. And notice the spots of the body you avoid. The thighs? The feet? Spend the most time there, as these are your bits that need the most love.

Sit for some time. I recommend 20 minutes. Why not use this time to do your meditation?

Rub off any excess oil with your oil towel, and then take a shower. Showering causes the pores to open, allowing the herbal oil to penetrate even deeper into the skin. You do not need to soap off the oil. The body will most likely absorb it all, especially if you are quite dry.

Make sure not to leave the oil on for more than 45 minutes, as this can actually clog the channels we are trying to cleanse. Also, make sure to use chemical-free, organic, cold-pressed oils. Do not use mineral oils such as baby oils.

Bathing Ritual

Traditionally in India, gods and goddesses are ritually bathed in the most nutritious foods and oils. As women, we can treat ourselves like a goddess by bathing in fine herbs, oils, and foods. Here are some decadent baths and nourishing scrubs that will leave your skin feeling as loved as a baby.

Pancha Amrit Snana—The Five Nectars Bath

- Ingredients: 2 tablespoons honey, 1 cup yogurt, 1 banana (mashed), ¼ cup sesame oil, 2 cups whole organic milk
- Combine all ingredients and mix until consistent throughout. Add to a warm bath, and soak for at least 20 minutes. Light candles. Play music.

Trinity Ava's Feel-the-Love Nourishing Sea Salt Body Scrub

Trinity Ava is one of my favorite herbal healer girlfriends. She is an accomplished herbalist, certified clinical aromatherapist, herbal marketing consultant, and teacher at the California School of Herbal Studies and Bastyr University. This is her recipe for a nourishing body scrub.

Needed:

1 clean, glass, wide-mouth pint (0.47 liter) jar

Preferably organic ingredients:
- 2 cups (473 ml) sea salt, coarse or fine
- 2 cups (500 ml) olive oil or sweet almond oil
- Essential oils: 10 drops lavender and 10 drops grapefruit
- (optional) 1 tablespoon finely ground rose petals

Preparation:

- Fill your clean jar with equal parts coarse and fine sea salt. If you prefer less texture to your scrub, use only fine-grain sea salt.
- Fill jar slowly with desired fatty oil, covering the salt with the oil. Cover jar with lid and shake well to evenly disperse the oil into the salt, or mix the salt and oil together with a chopstick or wooden tool. If you wish to use rose petals for color and aroma, add them to the salt and oil mixture and mix well. The rose petals are a beautiful addition to a traditional salt scrub, but they can be a bit messy for cleaning your shower or bathtub.
- Add 10 drops of lavender essential oil and 10 drops of grapefruit essential oil and mix well.

Optional essential oil favorites: vetiver, lime, ginger, Roman chamomile, ylang ylang, and red mandarin.

• • Essential Ideas • •

- Ayurvedic philosophy holds that the core nature of all reality is benign and beautiful. Our desire to be beautiful and radiant represents our desire to connect with the core essence of reality—beauty and love.
- Ayurvedic beauty is an inside-out and outside-in approach. Ayurvedic beauty says, "I am healthy and connected to life."
- With time and age, things tends to dry up. Rejuvenation is the practice of keeping things juicy. We call this rasayana, "the path of juice"!

Putting Ayurveda to Work

- Go to your bathroom and check out your products. Notice how many chemicals are in each product. Ditch as many unnatural products as possible.
- Stock your bathroom with this instead: neti pot, cold-pressed oils for your body type and season, sesame oil, rock salt or sea salt, tongue scraper, ghee, rose water, cucumber water, coconut oil, essential oils, and herbal powders. Once you've decided on your skin dosha, commit to preparing at least one of this chapter's all-natural skin product recipes. Use it for 40 days and note any changes both physically and emotionally, in regard to your skin.
- Get out your journal and write down how your skin feels this week—dry, oily, wrinkly, hot? Notice your skin tendencies and make a decision on which is your prominent skin dosha.

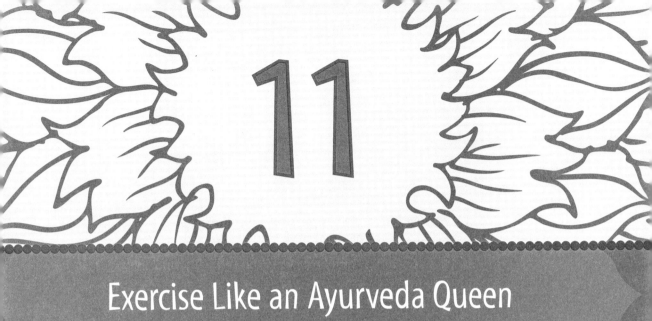

Exercise Like an Ayurveda Queen

e all know that exercise has incredible long-term health benefits. It can help you live longer, balance your weight, and boost your immune system. But what about the short-term effects of moving your body? What can exercise do to increase your happy-factor today? Both modern science and Ayurveda hold exercise as one of the most important of life's health-boosting, happy-inducing elixirs. And in a technology dependent world, sedentary lifestyles are leaving many of us feeling less then energized.

In fact, a significant amount of scientific research shows that exercise has a big effect on mood and well-being. Physical activity causes the brain to release endorphins—feel-good chemicals that promote feelings of happiness. Some researchers have found that moving the body on a daily basis can have a "large clinical impact" on the treatment of depression and anxiety, boosting general feelings of excitement and enthusiasm for life. One study even found that exercise was equally effective in treating depression as the commonly prescribed antidepressant medication Zoloft.[1]

So, it's clear that there is a direct link between your happiness and getting your hot body moving on a daily basis. But Ayurveda takes this exercise-happiness connection to a deeper level. You see, there is no one-size-fits-all in regard to exercise. When it comes to working out, Ayurveda takes dosha and season into account. And as an Ayurveda-inspired woman who understands her nature, you can tailor your exercise routines to honor your needs. With better insight into our mind/body tendency, we can work to bring ourselves into balance according to the type, frequency, and duration of our exercise routine. This chapter will teach you how you can best move your body for your type.

Vata Dosha

Think of some qualities of vata: cold, light, dry, rapid, changing, and mobile. Because of these inherent qualities, vata-type people will do best with forms of body movement that cultivate opposing qualities (i.e., warming, weight bearing, humid, slow, and steady). This kind of exercise will help relieve the muscle stiffness, anxiety, and tension associated with vata imbalance. It will also help get rid of any excess gas in the large intestine and colon and remove energetic blocks, allowing energy to move freely. Any body type will benefit from using the vata-reducing routine if the person is relatively healthy, and it is fall/early winter.

Tips for Exercising in a Way That Reduces Vata

Work with forms of exercise that are slow, steady, and even heavy. Weight lifting, slow-moving yoga, tai chi, long walks, hikes in nature, or mild biking are all good routines for reducing vata dosha.

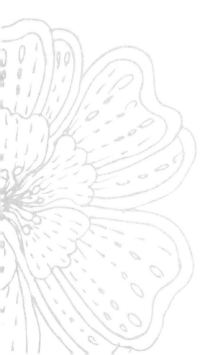

1. Vata types should work to a mild "glow," and should avoid dripping sweat. When we sweat, we detox, which is great, but too much sweat leads to a loss of ojas. If the sweat becomes sweet and silky, it means you have stopped detoxing and have moved into your life essence. Not good.
2. If practicing yoga, choose slow, steady classes over rapid power yoga. Moderately long holds and restorative yoga are also appropriate. Forward bends and twists in yoga reduce vata in the body and mind. When practicing, hug muscles to the bones for added support. Do not hold poses for too long, so as to avoid exhaustion.
3. Exercise slowly, with a calm and focused mind. Vata tends to get overly enthusiastic about exercise, overexert, and then quickly burn out. Focus on the long haul. Be a turtle, not a rabbit.

4. Try exercising in a way where you only breathe out of your nose. When you begin to pant out of mouth, you are taxing your heart. Stop, slow down, and rebuild. You will soon find that you can build up to longer and longer distances with only nose breathing. In this way, you slowly build cardiovascular health while not overtasking your cardiovascular and nervous systems.

5. Exercise with a breath that inhales all the way down to your roots. Breathe into your pelvic floor, lower back, and abdomen.

6. After exercising, make sure to rest. Take a *savasana* (corpse pose), even if you aren't practicing yoga.

Pitta Dosha

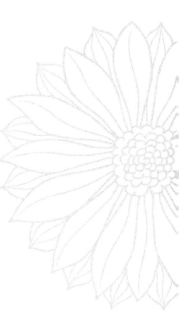

Remember some of the qualities of pitta: hot, light, oily, sharp, intense, and mobile. Because of these inherent qualities, pitta-type people will do best with forms of body movement that cultivate the opposing qualities (i.e., exercising in temperate or cool weather, and exercising in a calm and steady way). Working out in this manner will help relieve some of the tension, intensity, heat, and irritability associated with pitta imbalance. It will also help get rid of any excess Fire (i.e., stress and acid) in the body, most specifically in the sites where heat accumulates—small intestine, liver, blood, head, and eyes. If you exercise in a way that aggravates pitta, you will actually accumulate more Fire in those body parts. Any body type will benefit from using the pitta-reducing routine if they are relatively healthy and it is summer.

Tips for Exercising in a Way That Reduces Pitta

1. Work with forms of exercise that are slow, calming, and even cooling. Swimming, moderate biking, non-ambitious or non-competitive yoga, tai chi, long walks on the beach, hikes in nature, or mild biking are all good routines for pitta dosha.

2. Pitta types should work to a mild "glow," and should avoid dripping sweat. When we sweat, we detox, which is great, but

too much sweat leads to an increase in heat, which pitta types already have enough of. It also leads to a loss of ojas.

3. Pitta types are usually quite strong by nature. They can focus more on flexibility than strength.

4. Exercise in a way that feels fun, relaxed, and receptive. There is nothing that imbalances pitta more than an overly intense, competitive workout.

5. Emphasize mental calm over perfection of the craft. Try less, feel more. Cultivate a sense of receptivity and effortlessness, even as you exercise. Notice if you are in a self-critical or competitive state of mind.

6. If practicing yoga, choose calming, steady vinyasa classes over heated, power, or Bikram yoga. Moderately long holds and restorative classes are also appropriate. Forward bends, twists, and backbends on the belly are types of yoga poses that reduce pitta in the body and mind.

7. Try exercising in a way where you only breathe through your nose. Exercise with a breath that inhales all the way down to your low belly and hips, the center of water in the body.

8. After exercising, make sure to rest and cool down.

9. Pitta types can tend to be overly competitive and "burn out." Make sure to hydrate your pitta body with water or other liquids, particularly in the summer time.

Kapha Dosha

The qualities of kapha are cool, heavy, moist, slow, dull, and stagnant. Because of these inherent qualities, kapha-type people will do best with forms of body movement that cultivate the opposing qualities (i.e., warming, light, dry, quick, and mobile). Exercise done in this manner will help relieve some of the congestion and stagnation associated with this dosha, specifically in regard to getting rid of any excess phlegm and mucus in the chest and stomach. Kapha-reducing exercise will boost enthusiasm for life, stimulating us out of depression and lethargy. Any body type will benefit from using the kapha-reducing routine if the person is relatively healthy, and it is spring.

Tips for Exercising in a Way That Reduces Kapha

1. Work with forms of exercise that are quicker, energizing, and mildly heating. Quicker forms of yoga, jogging, biking, and jumping rope are all good routines.
2. Kapha can work up the biggest sweat of the three doshas.
3. Kapha types are usually strong by nature. They can focus more on flexibility and agility.
4. Exercise in a way that feels moving and dynamic. A little competition, speed, effort, and drive are actually good for kapha types.
5. Emphasize alertness and willpower.
6. If practicing yoga, choose forms that are more rapid and moving. Longer holds are also good for kapha, as they build intensity and circulation of blood and lymph. Backbends, yoga poses that stretch your side body, and twists are great for kapha types.
7. Try exercising in a way where you only breathe through the nose. Exercise with a breath that fills the entire chest cavity, including the back of the body.
8. After exercising, make sure to rest. But don't go lethargic. Kapha types have the tendency to overindulge in lounging around.

• • Essential Ideas • •

- Exercise, when done in the right way for your constitution, is Nature's instant happy pill.
- In general, all people will benefit from exercising in a way that balances seasonal energies. For example, if it's spring and you feel good, it's fun to do some kapha-reducing exercises, no matter what your type.
- If you are feeling any type of doshic imbalance, follow the exercise suggestions that help reduce that dosha. For example, if you

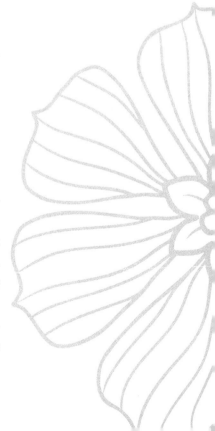

are feeling overheated and angry and have some acid indigestion, exercise in a way that reduces pitta, no matter the season.

Putting Ayurveda to Work

- Which form of exercise do you most often do? Is this the most balancing for your body?
- Reflect on how you can change up your exercise routine for the seasons.
- Sit for a moment and breathe into your belly. Tune in to what your body needs. Ask yourself, *Beautiful body, what form of exercise will best serve you today, or this week?* Wait for an answer. Commit to doing it.
- What can you do today to move your body? If you find you don't "have time" for a formal workout, can you walk to work, take the stairs instead of the elevator, or take a walk after dinner with your kids?

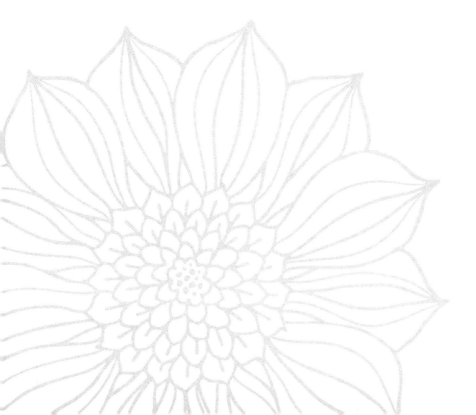

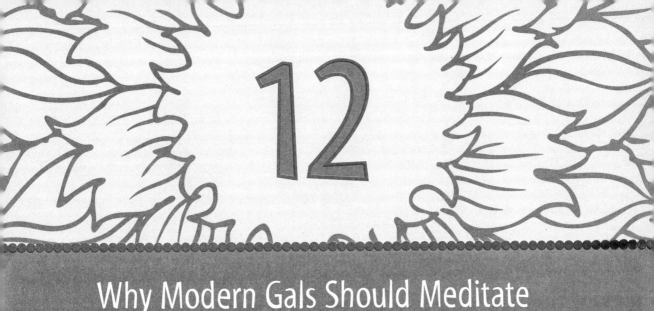

Why Modern Gals Should Meditate

One of the best ways to gain access to our soul and become truly happy is to practice sitting in silence. While diet and lifestyle changes definitely begin to reshape our energy and improve our wellness, it's meditation, and being able to feel our inner sensations, that really alter the deeper patterning in our minds. With time, a spiritual practice is what can catalyze big changes in our consciousness, and move us closer to our birthright—knowing who we really are.

About a decade ago, I was a young woman living alone in a foreign country, beginning to figure out who I was and what I wanted to do with my life. I had undergone several incredibly stressful events all around the same time—a divorce from my Spanish husband (my main connection to that foreign land); a change in jobs, from owning a ramshackle beach bar to working in a technology company with some

of the smartest people I'd ever met; and a solo move from one city in Spain to another.

In my new life of company dinners, marble mansions, and free-flowing champagne, I began having panic attacks. I'd never even heard of a panic attack before. I just thought I was dying. My boss at the time was also a somewhat shadily licensed psychologist (yes, the CEO of the tech company). He began giving me Valium. His exact words to me were, "You are probably just dehydrated and bored. You need to party more. Come out with us, have a few more drinks, and just have fun. All this panic attack stuff will blow over."

Thank God there was something in me that said, "Stop taking these pills. And stop drinking." I began praying. I prayed to Jesus, the God that had loved me as a little girl. I had heard yoga also helped calm you down, so I signed up for local classes a few weeks after trashing the Valium. That class saved me. I went to it almost every night for six months. Most of the classes ended with a short prayer and meditation. My panic attacks mostly subsided, and as I breathed into my body for perhaps the first time in my life, I felt something waking up inside of me—a force that I knew could, and would, eventually change me into who I was meant to become. A few years later, I found my current teacher, Yogarupa Rod Stryker, and I have been practicing meditation daily since our meeting.

I know my story probably isn't much different from yours. I know many women who claim that yoga saved their lives. But I believe meditation is our missing link to deeper healing. Plus, science has pretty much confirmed that meditation is a cure-all. Studies show that it has been successful in treating high blood pressure, heart disease, migraine headaches, autoimmune diseases, obsessive thinking, anxiety, depression, and hostility. It also has been shown to increase happiness, cause relaxation, augment our ability to pick up on the emotions of others, and improve attention and memory.[1] Why would anyone *not* want to meditate? I want to share a few of the techniques and practices I have learned from my lineage, and my own body's experience. These mediations were crucial in my own healing journey, and I know that they have the possibility to shape your experience as well.

The first thing to understand is that these meditations work from some core principles within Ayurvedic and yogic understandings. These principles are:

1. A lot of our misery comes from the unconscious stuff sitting beneath our surface thoughts.
2. Wherever your focus goes, energy flows.
3. When you focus your energy, your mind will get more quiet and focused, allowing you to see what is under the surface of your daily thoughts.
4. When you pull something up from your unconscious, it no longer has as much power over you.

5. Meditation eventually leads us to deeper and subtler layers of who we are. One of the deepest layers is called the *anandamaya kosha*—the body of bliss.

So, we meditate not just to get quiet, but also to experience inner bliss. If you close your eyes and get really quiet, you can feel that power starting to reveal itself. Seriously, close your eyes. Put your hand on your throat. Feel it? There is a pulse there—a kind of moving, vibrational quality of aliveness that doesn't feel totally physical. Just watching the ever-changing pulses in our bodies has the potential to open us to new inner experiences that melt fear and boost joy.

Keep going downward with your focus, and notice your belly. Do you feel alive, or is it dark or numb there? With time, you may start to notice that there is a wavelike beat in your belly. There is a secret rhythm sitting there, a gentle internal movement presence that, if accompanied by a sweet attitude of just watching, opens up inner chambers previously unvisited.

Like anything that really matters, meditation will take time and dedication. I find that many of the women I run across in my travels are stoked about the idea of meditation, but when it comes down to actually getting into it, there is resistance. While these practices are fairly simple, you will need to make them a priority if you want to truly experience transformation. No amount of spiritual study, workshop-hopping, or pondering the meaning of life whilst smoking a joint can really get you into the silence the way a daily meditation practice can. That is why I suggest that you pick one meditation and do it every day for at least 40 days. In this way, you will begin to connect with the fruits of practice that may not be as obvious

> **Love Makes Us Receptive to Change, with Special Guest Dr. Claudia Welch**
>
> *Almost every time my guru would put his students into meditation, he would say to do our practices lovingly, without thinking of them as a burden. He said this so often that I stopped hearing him. His words almost ceased to mean anything to me—until I was studying hormones and ran across this interesting fact: When we are in love, the hormone oxytocin increases. When oxytocin increases, it makes our brains more receptive to the creation of new neural pathways. And that comes in handy when we're trying to meditate and transform our thought patterns and perceptions.*
>
> ((For a complete version of Dr. Welch's piece on prana, meditation, and unraveling old patterns, check out www.healthyhappysexylife.com.)

from one practice to the next. It is also a good idea to keep a journal of your daily meditation.

Meditate Like an Ayurveda Queen

When you think of meditation, you may see an image of a bald-headed Buddha, sitting, spine erect under a droopy-limbed tree, attempting to calm his mind by watching his thoughts. This is an excellent approach to getting the mind quiet. But there are other, more Tantric techniques for accessing our silent power. Rather than focusing on thoughts, witnessing them, or trying to stop them, we can deeply feel and see the sensations in our own body.

The body is like a temple, and when we meditate, we walk into it with reverence and awe. In the temple, you can give yourself permission to deeply feel and follow your sensations as portals. Your sensations and internal experiences become the juice for your imagination. In a way, you will make your own inner body so darn interesting that the mind has no choice but to focus on that silent beauty. In other words, we give the mind a job. And that job is to create the most rad internal atmosphere, like an Inner Eden, for the soul to experience itself. In this Tantric approach, you will know your meditation is working when you begin to feel more and more in love.

Meditation for Gathering Your Fire

Use this meditation for more energy, power, and transformational capacity. It is also beneficial when you need to know the answer to an important question or make a decision. It reconnects us to our gut feeling and helps us gather the power necessary for accomplishing our goals, both worldly and spiritual. Try working with this practice for at least 40 days, for 15–45 minutes daily.

Close your eyes and let your body relax and settle as you sit with your spine tall and long. Feel your spine lengthen with the inhalation, and feel the navel draw in toward the spine with the exhalation. Allow

Meditation: An Instant Feel-Good Pill

The benefits of meditation are irrefutable. Regular meditation has been scientifically shown to reduce stress and anxiety, depression, chronic pain, insomnia, menstrual issues, and migraine headaches. It also helps boost the immune system, deepen restful sleep, and reduce aging. Studies show that meditation can even increase self-esteem as it triggers the "feel-good" chemicals in the body, enhancing right-brain (initiative and connective) function.[2]

your spine to be tall, yet relax the muscles alongside it. Begin by internally witnessing the navel move in as you breathe out, and the chest expand as you breathe in. Do this for 1 minute. Now, begin to smooth and even out your inhale and exhale.

Slowly begin to feel the temperature of the air at your nostrils. Begin to quietly witness the touch of your breath as it enters into the nostrils and then leaves them again. Do this for a few minutes. Thoughts may rise and fall. The idea is not to empty out the mind, but to watch its contents with a sense of nonattachment.

Now, begin to watch the same air rise from the tip of your nostrils to the middle of your brain. Visualize a line of light, or feel the energy that rides alongside your breath entering your nostrils, touching the middle of your brain, and leaving as you exhale. Visualize this light of breath as a golden elixir, connecting you to the innate energy of the Divine One.

The nature of our deepest energy and power is one of love and expansion. After a while, you may feel this light in your midbrain as a pulse or a vibration that wants to expand and love you. Allow this golden elixir to move down your body slowly, through the spine. Allow this light to take its time to reach the point of your belly button, just inside the spine.

Let this golden elixir become established at the navel. See it building into a vibrant flame—a robust, living, powerful expression of who you are, of your highest power and capacity. Feel that you are connecting to the part of you that has sparked every moment of active love, courage, and inspiration in your life. For 1–2 minutes, just allow your whole being to be absorbed into the Fire of your internal power and capacity. Whatever arises—joy, doubt, a feeling of *Am I doing this right?*—can be thrown into the visualization of Fire at the belly. Stay in this presence as long as you like. Now would be a good time to begin to chant a mantra into the energetic Fire connection you have created at your belly. If you need a mantra, choose one from the following section of this chapter.

To come out of the meditation, simply lower your head to your heart, offering gratitude for the practice, and slowly begin to come back.

> ### Meditate with Me at Home
>
> It's much easier to become steeped in these practices when you have a recording to follow. I have created some online, audible versions of these meditations. You can find them at www.healthyhappysexylife.com.

Meditation for a Broken Heart

Use this meditation for healing your heart. This meditation brings more self-esteem, self-love, and self-healing into the body. It builds our connection to nourishing energy, associated with our ability to take from the outside in. This type of energy gets depleted when we feel heartbroken and unloved, or when we experience sensory overload from the world outside.

You can do this meditation sitting down, but I find it helpful to lie down with some support under my spine, such as a folded blanket or a bolster. I find that the heart can heal easier when it feels the earth below holding it and softening it.

Close your eyes and let your body relax and settle into its connection to the earth. Feel that you are in a nurturing, soothing place, and that you are fully safe to relax. For a few minutes, notice the simple miracle of your breath. The inhale raises the navel center away from you, without you trying, and the exhale lowers the belly back onto you. Again, try not to try. Simply watch your belly as you become more and more relaxed.

Now, begin to smooth and even out the breath. Take a few minutes to get the inhale and exhale as smooth and even as possible. The more relaxed you become, the subtler the breath may become. Now begin to quietly witness the sensation of your breath as it enters the nostrils and then leaves the nostrils. Do this for a few minutes. Thoughts may rise and fall. The idea is not to empty out the mind, but to watch its contents with a sense of nonattachment.

Now begin to watch the same air rise from the tip of your nostrils to the middle of your brain. Relax and visualize a line of light, or feel the energy that rides alongside the breath entering the nostrils, touching the middle of your brain, and leaving as you exhale. Visualize this light of breath as a golden elixir, connecting you to the innate energy of the Divine One. After a while, you may feel this light in your midbrain as a pulse or a vibration that wants to expand and love you. Allow this golden elixir to move down your body slowly to your heart—the center of your chest, about 4–5 inches below your collarbone. You can even place your hand on your heart, if it helps you connect to this center of love and spiritual insight.

As you breathe in again, feel this light move from your midbrain to your heart; as you breathe out, feel your breath permeate your heart with presence, dissolving and resolving any stuck energy there. As you breathe in, sense a golden, honey-like light drawing from the midbrain into the space of your heart. As you breathe out, see this golden elixir seating itself in the very center of your heart. Keep repeating. With every inhale, lovingly pull this honey-light from the midbrain to the heart, and as you exhale, seat this light in the center of your body at the level of the heart.

As you continue with this visualization, you may notice that there are some spots in your chest that feel sadness, pain, stickiness, tightness, loneliness, anger, or any other sensation or emotion that is not vast and loving.

When you find these spots, you can see them as blockages sitting on the vast open field of your heart. Let your awareness stay in these spots, and keep breathing in the golden light, allowing your attention and love to penetrate the dark corners of your heart. Remember, energy follows focus. The more you can soften into love and send your focus to the stickiness, the greater the chance that the blockage can dissolve and resolve itself. Keep moving your awareness through the visualization, and allowing the energy to open and disperse any blocks in the heart.

Finally, there may come a moment when the heart is just so full of light and openness that you can abandon the technique and simply enjoy breathing into the new space of the heart. Now would be a good time to begin to chant a mantra into the energetic heart connection you have created. There's more on mantras in the next section.

To come out of the meditation, simply deepen your breath, offering gratitude for the practice. Slowly begin to move your body and come back.

Meditation for Grounding and Letting Go

Use this meditation for connecting to the energy of grounding and letting go into Mama Earth. This meditation reduces anxiety and increases our capacity to let go of toxicity, whether it be bad relationships, illness, stress, or emotional baggage. It is highly stabilizing, cooling, and calming for the mind and body, and helps boost our sense of belonging to the Earth-tribe in which we live.

You can do this meditation sitting down, but I find it helpful to lie down with some support under the spine, such as a folded blanket or a bolster. Sometimes I can feel a deeper connection to the energy of surrender when I can feel the earth below me. Try working with this practice for at least 40 days, 15–45 minutes daily.

Close your eyes and let your body relax and settle into its connection to the earth. Feel that you are in a nurturing, soothing place, and that you are fully safe to relax. Notice for a few minutes the simple miracle of your breath. The inhale raises the navel center away from you, without you trying, and the exhale lowers the belly back onto you. Again, try not to try. Simply watch your belly as you become more and more relaxed.

Begin to smooth and even out the inhale and exhale. Take a few minutes to get the inhale and exhale as smooth and even as possible. The more relaxed you become, the subtler the breath may become.

Slowly begin to bring your attention into the base of your spine, the root center. As you feel your body inhale, allow your whole pelvic floor to relax, let go and expand. Sense that your inhale can literally expand your cervix and perineum. As you feel your body exhale, engage the pelvic floor muscles upward, gently pulling them in and up toward your belly. As you inhale, completely relax them, but do so as smoothly and slowly as possible. Stay very attuned to the inhale and the relaxing of the pelvic floor in particular. It is in this moment where we surrender and let go, grounding into the earth. As you exhale and engage the muscles, sense that you are drawing in the qualities of stability and rootedness. Do these pulsations slowly 8–10 times.

After the pulsations, relax and let go of all effort. As you inhale, draw all of yourself—your feelings, your attention—to the root of your spine. As you exhale, feel all physical and mental toxins leaving the body through the base of the spine, out into the core of the earth, which is Fire. That Fire can digest anything. Repeat this visualization 10 times.

Now, see and feel, or have the intention to see and feel, a downward-facing dark blue triangle at the base of your spine. See its base at the level of your low belly, hips, and groin. See the tip of the triangle at the base of your spine, pointing downward into the earth. Feel and see energy moving downward as bright and beautiful flashes of lightning. Hear the sound of static electricity as you ground this lightning out of the root of your spine and into the core of the earth. Feel a powerful sense of being grounded and stable. Stay with this part of practice for 5-10 minutes. Notice how seeing and hearing enable the sense of groundedness to increase.

Finally, there may come a moment when you feel such a connection to the earth, as well as your own downward, letting-go capacities, that you can abandon the technique and meditate on this force of surrender. Now would be a good time to begin to chant a mantra into the energetic earth connection you have created. There's more on mantras in the next section.

To come out of the meditation, simply deepen your breath, offering gratitude for the practice. Slowly begin to move your body and open your eyes.

Meditation for Gathering and Expanding Your Energy

This energizing practice brings clarity and focus as you learn to collect your life-force energy. This practice helps us gather the energy we need for both spiritual and worldly goals. To begin, close your eyes and let your body relax. For a few minutes, notice the simple miracle of your breath. Your inhale raises the navel center away from you, without you trying, and the exhale lowers the belly back down. Again, try not to try. Simply watch your belly as you become more and more relaxed.

Now, bring your awareness to your nostrils and begin to smooth and even out your inhale and exhale. Take a few minutes to get the inhale and exhale as smooth and even as possible, feeling the texture and temperature of the way the air moves through your nostrils, from the tip to the bridge of the nose. Feel the current of air rising and falling along the ceiling of the nostril. Spend some time here, just feeling the ceiling of the nostril. The more effortless you become, the more you will feel that you aren't controlling or shaping the breath. The breath is breathing itself. The more you relax, the more you will sense that there is subtle energy that precedes and follows the breath. This is your connection to prana.

Focus on this connection, at the ceiling of the nostril, into the midbrain. You may sense a presence or light. Feel light pulling breath in and out of you. The nature of this light is expansion. Feel this light move into your midbrain. With time, the brain will almost feel as if it's bathing in light. When you sense or feel light, let go of all techniques and simply rest in the luminous light of the mind. You are now in a place of "gathering" or "collecting energy." Now would be a good time to begin to chant a mantra into the pranic presence you have created.

To come out of the meditation, simply deepen your breath, offering gratitude for the practice. Slowly begin to move your body and come back into the world with an energized spirit.

Mantra

What is *mantra*? The Sanskrit root *man* means "mind" or "to think." The word *tra* comes from the root word for "to protect, guide, or lead." So a mantra is a sound, vibration, or *bhav* (feeling or meaning) that protects, guides, and leads the mind. Mantra can also be translated as "mind protector." Another meaning of mantra is "a measure," as in a vibration or rhythm that we attune to, instead of the normal patterning (and therefore vibration) of the untamed mind. According to Rolf Sovik, author of *Moving Inward: The Journey to Meditation*, "A mantra is an audible form of pure consciousness—a pure note reaching the mind from the silent interior space of consciousness. Through meditation, the sound of that note is awakened in the mind, transforming inner life by its presence."[3]

Why Use a Mantra?

I once heard a respected meditation teacher say that a mantra acts like a cleaning force—a subtle but extremely strong broom that sweeps the basement of your subconscious. I like to think of using mantra as a way of tuning into a different music station. So often throughout the day, we subject ourselves to an endless stream of mind chatter. Studies show that most of the thoughts we have today are dramatically similar to the thoughts we had yesterday. A mantra helps us shift that old thought-flow and tune our attention to higher vibrations of love, compassion, power, and capacity. A mantra is also a challenge. It is like Fire. When you use a mantra to challenge your old patterning, you create an internal Fire. That Fire melts the old patterning, opening you up for new possibilities and perspectives on your life.

How to Work with a Mantra

You may already have a mantra from a teacher or a tradition you are working with, or you may choose one of the mantras I offer in this book. We look at the practice of using a mantra as working from the gross to the more subtle realms. First, begin by saying your mantra out loud. With time, sometimes as little as a few minutes, you may be able to move into saying your mantra quietly, like a whisper. Then, after a few minutes, try saying it silently to yourself. You may work with this layer of mantra repetition for a few weeks, or even years. With time, you may begin to actually hear your mantra beginning to unfold on its own. This is a good sign that you are surrendering to the power and vibration held in this sacred sound. Maintain your awareness as a listener of the mantra. There may be 10 percent of you holding the mantra, or having the intention to hear the mantra, and 90 percent of you just listening. With time and practice, the subtlest levels of the mantra will emerge. There may come a time when you do not hear the words at all, but a visceral pulse of the mantra begins to emerge. It may manifest in more and more subtle ways—as light or symbol or even the apparition of a god or goddess image. Keep connecting to the sacred pulse of the mantra, letting it dissolve and resolve any and all obstruction, bringing you back into the silent roar of love at your heart. With time, the mantra is no longer said or heard; it begins to say you. You become the mantra.

It's important to receive a mantra that has been empowered, or held, by a lineage or tradition. Anyone can go online, Google "mantra," and start chanting. But the true sacred power of a mantra comes in its being held in love, by a teacher, for many years. In this way, the mantra is "unlocked." The following mantras are transformative mantras, empowered, and given to you by my teachers, a lineage in the Himalayan yoga tradition.

Om—The sound of everything. The sound of Universal consciousness and creation.

So Ham [SO-HUM] "I am That. I exist." I translate So Ham as, "I am the very thing I keep looking for." It is the universal sound of both being and becoming. *So* is the sound of an inhale. *Ham* is the sound of exhale. As I inhale, I hear and am Universal Being. As I exhale, I hear myself merging the individual into the Everything, the Goodness, the Highest Power.

Aum tryambakam yajamahe sugandhim pushti vardhanam urvarukamiva bandhanan mrityor mukhsiya mamritat—the *Mahamrityun Jaya* mantra.

Phonetic translation (for English speakers): Om tree-um-buh-kuhm yuh-jaa-muh-hey | soo-gan-dheem poosh-ti var-dhuh-num | oor-vaar-oo-kuhm ivuh buhn-duh-naahn | mrut-yoor mook-sheeya maa-mru-taaht.[4]

This is a traditional healing mantra, its vibrations sending out ripples of healing wisdom, strength, and willpower into the mind and body. When we meditate on this mantra, we are calling forth the Divine inside and outside of us for protection. We call out to that which is intrinsically beautiful, to that which brings delight.

The mantra says: "I call out to everything that is beautifully sweet and fragrant in life, like the delicate aroma that a Jasmine flower releases effortlessly. I call upon my Inner Teacher to guide me like a skillful gardener who helps me grow. May this skillful gardener, just as She unravels the vines that choke the other plants, teach me how to untangle myself from my own attachments, fears, and illnesses, so that I may know my true Heart. May She unravel any vines on my Heart of Hearts."

Use this mantra to connect with the healer within. It is particularly potent for a teacher, mother, doctor, therapist, gardener, cook, herb-maker, or anyone dedicated to enlivening their highest well-being. This mantra is literally the Victorious Mantra, offering victory over "the great death."

Om bhur, bhuvah, svahtat savitur varenyambhargo devasya dhimahidhiyo yo nah prachodayat—Gayatri mantra.

Phonetic translation (for English speakers): Om Bhoor Bhoo-va-ha Swa-ha | tut sa-vee-toor var-ey-eyn-yum | bhar-go day-vuhs-yuh dhee-muh-hee | dhee-yo yo nuh pracho-die-yaat.[5]

This mantra comes to us from the *Rig Veda*, one of the oldest religious texts on the planet. The word *gayatri* means "She who protects the singer" (from *gai*, "to sing," and *trai*, "to protect"). With this mantra we call upon our Divine Mother, asking for her protection as we move through the obstacles of life.

This mantra says, "Oh Divine Light inside of me, Oh radiant one, I meditate on you, like the most adorable Sun of my spiritual consciousness. May you wake me up."

• • Essential Ideas • •

- We meet our soul by sitting in our own silence.
- A mantra helps us connect to that living silence. It is a sacred sound vibration that guides, protects, and expands the mind.
- Working with a mantra helps us move out of the thoughts and stories we normally tell ourselves, giving us more freedom to experience truth.
- The health and happiness benefits of meditation are irrefutable. Try one of the meditations in this book for at least 40 days to feel the benefits. You can get an audible recording of these practices at www.healthyhappysexylife.com.

Putting Ayurveda to Work

The Perfect Meditative Day: Start your morning with one of the meditations above. Practice it for 5 minutes to begin. Work up to 20–45 minutes daily. Use a mantra from the list in this chapter. Repeat it silently 54–108 times. In the afternoon, do a recorded yoga nidra practice, lying down. You can find an audible recording of yoga nidra at www.healthyhappysexylife.com.

Create your own meditation practice for the next 40 days. You can do it! In your journal, write about your experiences after each seated session.

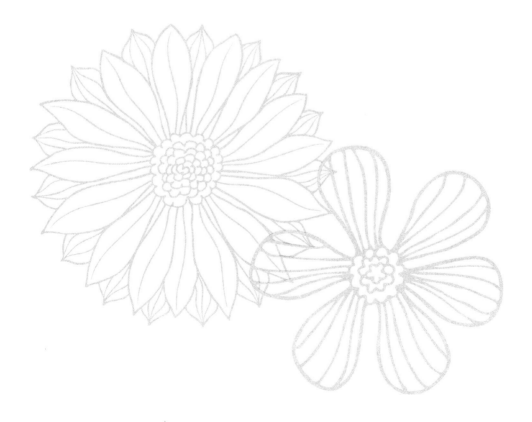

Part IV

Sexy

S-E-X. This tiny three-letter word stirs up so much inside a girl. From elation to trauma, pleasure to shame, whatever your beliefs or experiences, sex is a superpower. It's got charge. And that charge ain't going anywhere soon. In fact, the ancient scriptures speak of sex as the strongest force on the material plane. When used for good, it is a wellspring of the highest pleasure. When misused, it can become a breeding ground for manipulation, attachment, and spiritual backtracking. This section of the book is a love offering, based on the wisdom Ayurveda has instilled into my own healing journey around sexuality. I will admit, it wasn't the easiest chapter to write. I am no Dr. Ruth, and my own journey into sexuality and intimacy is far from being complete. But without addressing the third pillar of a woman's health—her sexuality—we would miss out on the life-spring of our deep happiness and vitality.

Sex lies at the core of our existence. Everywhere we look women (and men) are hungry for more pleasure and a deeper fulfillment in the sexual realm. Our media culture bombards us with images of women having orgasms over shampoo, or men who woo with expensive watches and cars. This same bombardment of images is matched by a decline in wisdom around real intimacy and quality sex. Luckily, we have Ayurveda's deep wisdom surrounding this sensuous, often-misunderstood aspect of our existence. Ayurveda promises us that the primal life force of sex, when channeled correctly and used wisely, can be a power source that helps us on the path toward enlightenment, fulfillment in relationships, procreation, creativity, and healing.

My Own Sexy Evolution

Like many women in American culture, I grew up seeing fad diets, boob jobs, eyebrow waxes, pedicures, and bleach-blond highlights. I also come from a long family lineage of beauty-seeking, charm-schooling, Southern-belle women. My mama was a high school beauty queen. One of my cousins is a famous hair and makeup artist who was so beautiful that she actually chopped off all her hair so men would leave her alone in the grocery store. In my family, if you are a woman, you were taught that the "sexy factor" is an important part of your worth. My story may not be that different from yours.

But these "sexy regimes," while not inherently wrong, didn't fulfill my heart or satiate my sexual desires. I was confused. I was taught to try to be sexy, but at the same time to hide my sexuality. I was supposed to be pretty but ashamed of my deeper desires for intimate connection and physical experiences. This conflicting messages totally deflated my self-esteem. I could never be sexy or beautiful enough to fit the media model, and at the same time, my true sexual essence remained asleep.

Practicing Ayurveda and yoga began to wake me up to what was hidden inside. Something started stirring inside my belly—a pulsing, a longing to feel alive, a need to vibrate with the rhythm of music, to suck on a purple plum until the sticky juices ran down my chin, to smell the mineral-rich dirt in my backyard, to breathe in cold air on a snowy, moonlit night. I wanted to be able to touch my thighs without cringing, pushing into my cellulite as if to say, "Mama, you are so fleshy, and that is fine." I wanted to feel that I had permission to be a sexual creature with every one of my five senses.

When I learned the wisdom of Ayurveda, I felt that I had tapped into a stream of knowledge that honored life itself as something inherently sexual. Every cell in your body makes love to itself and multiplies. Why would you be anything less than a sexual goddess?

In this section, we will work to restore, heal, and empower our sacred female center—the womb. In this way, we can clear the way for the awe of sexual ecstasy to flow naturally. We will also approach sexuality from the perspective that views making love as taking many forms, whether personal or with a partner. The gateways of the five senses will be used as portals for developing our sensuality and happiness in the sexual realm. In this sense, it makes no difference whether you are in a relationship or not. In fact, this chapter is more about connecting to the tremendous charge of your own life force than the latest-and-greatest sex position or aphrodisiac (although those are nice as well). I can't wait for this section to make love to you.

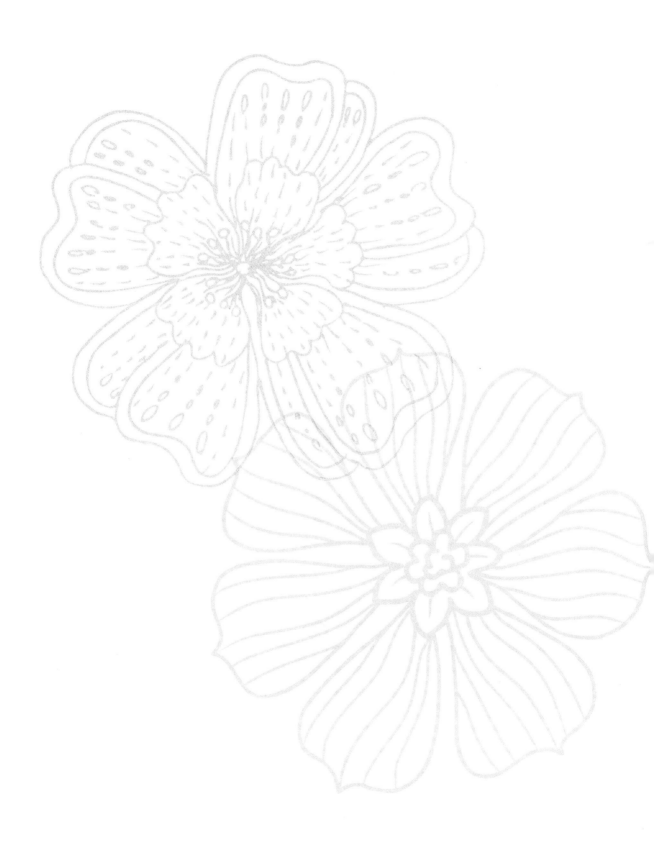

13

Ayurveda Sexuality and Deep Female Vitality

Remember Ayurveda's three pillars of health—food, sleep, and sexual energy? These pillars refer to the deep need we all have for nourishment, rest, and creativity. And the health of your female sexuality is just as important as any dietary or sleep practice for maintaining a healthy body, an eased mind, and a connection to your vitality. Our sexuality is a force in all of us that longs to be channeled and intimately experienced.

Sexual Nutrition

Kama shakti can be translated as "pleasure-power." In order to learn how to build our kama shakti, think about sexual energy and its physical, sensual expression as you would think about food. Just as we want to have the proper amounts and types of foods at specific times of day, we can also think of sexuality as a form of multilevel emotional nutrition.

Let me give an example: Rarely is a huge slice of cheesecake at midnight a good idea. But there are those rare occasions when a girl needs a midnight snack, and so on this unique and unlikely occasion, it may even be beneficial to veer off track. Similarly, rarely is a quickie in the airplane bathroom a nourishing, emotionally gratifying experience. That said, once in a while, racking up frequent flyer miles in the Mile High Club could be fun and exhilarating. Still, nobody likes plane food after the first few exciting trips, if ya get my drift. The bottom line is that too little or repressed sexuality leads to emotional emaciation, lack of nurturance, or perversion, while too much sex can lead to exhaustion, both physically and mentally, especially if we are having sex that is not connected to deep love. Our kama shakti is built around having awareness about what is nourishing for us in regard to how, when, and where we express our sex power.

We can cultivate deeper sexual fulfillment by using Ayurvedic principles. Ayurveda helps us align our sexuality with the natural pulls of time, environment, and personal needs, as well as nurturing a sense of *bhavana*, meaning "intention" and "deep feeling." Sexual expression, done with the right intention, can bring more love and intimacy into the world. In fact, sex is even more potent than food because of the intensity of its energetic build. Expressed with the proper intention, our sexuality has the power to boost our feelings of intimacy with the world, as well as awaken the dormant, life-giving energy inside all of us. Just as the silence of meditation brings about shifts in consciousness and energetic alterations, sexual expression can also momentarily shift us out of mundane mind patterns and into the sublime bliss of the eternal.

Sex and the Three Doshas

Before looking at sex in relation to the doshas, let's be clear: We are all a composite of all three doshas. There are times when you may feel like making love like a bunny (vata style) or lounging about like a tigress (kapha style). Remember, you have all of nature's gifts at your disposal, so don't put yourself in a sexual doshic box.

That said, we do have tendencies that we were born with, and those tendencies lead us toward behaviors, which in turn have their own doshic expressions. For example, vata is the part of our sexual expression that is mobile. When vata is balanced, we have freedom of movement, but also the ability to hold back our climax. When out of balance, climax can happen too fast and sex can leave us feeling depleted and breathless. Pitta is the part of our sexuality that relates to sexual vitality and vigor. It is the part of us that initiates sex and feels the burning passion for our lover. When out of balance, we may have no desire. Kapha sexuality is related to our sexual staying power, potency, and physical unctuousness. When in balance, our sex secretions are of good quantity and quality. Excess kapha can lead to sexual laziness and a heavy quality to lovemaking.

Sexual expression is all about expansiveness. Through the union of two beings, and orgasm, there is a potentiality to experience a state of consciousness very different from the consciousness you hold, say, in line at the post office or on the phone with your mother (thank God). Due to this potential for expansion, sex can be incredibly healing or incredibly destructive.

Healthy, life-bringing, satisfying sex requires open channels. Think of the entire mind/body as a complex, an interrelated system of physical and energetic tubes (*srotas* and *nadis*). Just as there are channels that move our blood, lymph, and waste products, there are also channels that move our sexual energy. In general, if we are blocked in any of the channels, our sexual energy can be blocked. This is why chronically constipated women commonly suffer from depressed libido and sleep disorders, in that both sleep and sex require a relaxing and an opening in the channels that govern letting go.

Similarly, if we are worried or unsatisfied, our sex channels get blocked. In this holistic framework, taking care of your digestion, skin, and emotions can create a mandala-like positive effect on every other realm of your life. Who would have thought it? Igniting the power of your digestion may be the best way to have more fulfilling orgasms. Let's learn some ancient sage wisdom on how we can enhance healthy sexuality.

Boosting Our Pleasure-Power— Kama Shakti

What is pleasure-power? Pleasure-power has everything to do with cultivating our ability to feel and experience pleasure in daily life—in and out of the bedroom. It's about getting quiet and content enough to experience the immense beauty that is always present when our senses are tuned in.

There are many ways to build this pleasure-power. When we use the basic principles of Ayurveda, we will undoubtedly have enhanced sexual vitality. Specifically, the text says that we will "get stimulated like a bull." And while I kind of love the idea of being as potent as a beefy bull, we should be aware that Ayurveda is not only referring to our increased ability to successfully ignite our partner's flame, but also an increased strength and vitality to create in the world, whether that be birthing a baby, becoming a doctor, or knitting a scarf.

Throw your women's magazines straight into the trash, because here are Ayurveda's aphrodisiac techniques for boosting your pleasure-power:

- Anoint yourself and your beloved with fine oils—when was the last time you were anointed?
- Massage your beloved. Receive massages from your beloved.
- Perfume your body. Chemical perfumes do not stimulate the sexy vixen within. Find an all-natural scent such as jasmine or honeysuckle. Give a musky scent to the man in your life.
- Take a bath. If it can be outdoors, even better.
- Be beautiful. It is said that there is no better aphrodisiac than pure beauty. And this is not related to any particular beauty standard, but refers to the lustrous radiance of healthy skin, clean body parts, bright eyes, clean nails and groomed hair.
- Better your digestion and elimination. It's hard for a person with chronic constipation to feel sexy. Similarly, chronic pitta leads to strong breath, body odor, and skin rash. Chronic kapha brings about a heaviness to the personality and a sluggish demeanor. By cleaning up our doshic imbalances, we clear the channels for sexual expansion.
- Wear a garland. This may sound outlandish (or just Hawaiian), but women in India today still walk around, conducting their daily business, with decadent streams of intoxicating jasmine flowers in their hair. What would the Western world feel like if women suddenly decided to drape their bodies in orchids at the office?
- Hear adorations. We build our sexual potency by being adored. If you are single, it doesn't matter—the adorations can come from any loved one in your life.

- Create a clean, comfortable living space. There is nothing that kills the creative mood quicker than dust bunnies and old cartons of take-out. Clutter and hoarding dampen libido.
- Buy flowers. Flowers are the sexual organs of plants. Having them in your bedroom will entice sexual longings.
- Invest in fine bedding and soft clothing. The ancients knew how important thread count and buttery-feeling clothing were for sensual feelings. My motto: 'Tis better one cashmere sweater than a closet full of fake fabrics.
- Hear the chirping of happy birds. The fact that we don't have enough happy birds in our bedroom windowsills may be related to why stressed-out city folks have less sex drive. If you can't house birds, then spend more time in nature.
- Wear things that tinkle and sparkle. There is something so sensual about the clinking of a woman's bangles as she goes about her tasks. Apparently, men in ancient India used to go wild for the sound of a gal's bracelets. Sigh. Those were the days.
- Walk, talk, and breathe with yourself or your beloved, in nature. Sometimes just a moonlit walk can shift us into the ambitionless, pleasure-experiencing side of our brain.
- Indulge your beloved with sweet speech. Save the, "Honey, can we talk?" conversations for later. To stoke desire, sit together in silence and breathe, or lie down together and just stay present to the miracle of your beloved's breath.
- Shift your expectation around outcomes. It may be more fulfilling to think of your partner not as someone who will go off on a hunt to bring you your pleasure, but as a witness to or participant in the unfolding of your pleasure from within. In the throes of passion, it can be transformative to get a little distance between the act of flesh and blood and the soul that exists inside the body. Pay homage and respect to the soul-jewel that lies in your arms. This is a doorway into deep love and deeper sexuality. If you are single, you can still practice appreciating others in your life for who they are—seeing their beauty without regard for outcome.[1]

Let Your Five Senses Take You There

Sometimes our mechanical, technological, scheduled world is simply not sexy. There is nothing mysterious about having to pencil in sexual encounters with your husband into an overbooked day planner (although it's better than not connecting at all). Moreover, while high-speed internet allows us nearly uninterrupted connectivity, studies show that the more we use the internet, the more disconnected we feel from our loved ones. Ayurveda offers incredible tools for strengthening the five senses, moving us back into the realm of the sensual before we lose touch with it completely. Many studies are looking into the reality of how internet use garbles our brain, disrupting our sensitivity to pleasure from subtle sources. Nicholas Carr, author of *The Shallows: What the Internet is Doing to Our Brain*, states, "The internet is an interruption system. It seizes our attention only to scramble it."[2] One key way we connect to our sensuality is through the power of focus. As technology continues to reduce this capacity, we are left hungry for the real nurturance that comes from a calm, focused mind perceiving the beauty of the world. Honing the senses refines the pleasure-power, leading to a boost of sensuality in daily life, as well as a deeper appreciation for the outside world.

Let's start with touch. We can keep the channels of our skin alive and receptive to the tactile by massaging it daily with warm oil (see chapter 9). When the skin channels are not blocked or dry, they are able to better perceive and receive the subtle energy emanating from the heart of those we love (children, lover, Grandma, pet gerbil), as well as our own heart. To boost your tactile receptors, practice giving and receiving loving or even sensual touch as a meditation. Ask your friend or partner to slowly run his hands over your skin. Meditate on the feeling of being touched.

Sight is important for expanding our creative capacity and appetite for life. The sense of sight is not only related to what your optometrist tells you at your annual eye visit. It is also related to our ability to observe the world, as well as ourselves, with awareness. In the pleasure-power context, this is about picking up on the subtle—a shift in your partner's gaze, a change in their expression, a soft movement of hand to face. The importance of sight to sexuality may be why we get ticked off if our partner doesn't notice our new hair cut. It's not about the highlights or the new dress; it's about the fact that the Divine Feminine wants to be seen. The more you develop your subtle powers of sight, the more you will spontaneously and deeply see your loved ones. They will also feel more seen by you. Enhancing our ability to stay present while lovingly observing the world boosts sexual energy more than any beauty product ever can. Practice "deep seeing." Pick an object of beauty (preferably one that is not moving much)—a blooming cherry blossom tree, the pattern on top of your next latte, a snowcapped mountain—and simply look at it. Spend at least 5 minutes gazing at your beauty-object. Notice what subtle patterns and colors emerge. Notice how this deep-seeing practice affects your own mind and heart.

Smell has a lot to do with sexual attraction. Maintaining a proper diet and lifestyle will enhance your smell, making your body the most irresistible perfume on the market. There is nothing less sexy than last night's lamb kabob covered up by cologne of some kind. And if your loved one comes to you with a noxious-fume-emitting armpit situation, you don't need to immediately send him packing. Ayurveda offers many ways that we can actually alter our smells by cleansing and using spices as medicines. Fenugreek does wonders for body smells and makes your vaginal fluids smell and taste sweet! To spice up your bedroom, consider giving the linens a light mist with jasmine or vetiver essential oil hydrosols. The smell of natural elements is a huge aphrodisiac—open your windows and let in the smell of fresh rain, wet earth, or salty air. Studies show that men are most attracted to smells that are related to food (what a shock). The top of the list? Vanilla. Hilariously, "Cinnabon" and "pumpkin pie" were a close second.[3]

Our minds are our biggest sexual organs, so sweet nothings whispered into our ears will definitely build sexual energy. But Ayurveda encourages us to think a little broader. To be a turned-on woman, Ayurveda asks us to tune in to the sounds of Nature in general. The chirping of crickets, a flowing creek, children's laughter, the musical cacophony of a busy subway line, our favorite symphony—by being in tune with sounds, we train our ears to become life-appreciating, life-worshipping organs.

Taste can be enhanced by savoring life more fully. Often we rush through meals so fast that we don't allow ourselves to actually taste the food. We do the same with our sexual energy. In fact, it's not a stretch to say that we can determine much about the state of our own sexual energy by our relationship to tasting food. You can also tell a lot about someone else's sensual style by observing their relationship to cooking and eating. I once had a boyfriend who was a chef. Before I decided whether or not we would be lovers, I watched him in the kitchen. The way he skillfully chopped vegetables and slowly tasted everything left my knees weak. He taught me that enjoying food slowly and with awareness translated into the ability to slow down in the bedroom.

Sacred Sensual Sleep Chamber

Whether you are coupled or single, straight or gay, young or old, setting the scene for sensuality is another key way we boost sexual energy flow. There is nothing that kills the mood faster than a TV or a buzzing mini-fridge in your lovemaking and sleep chamber. "Hey, honey, there's a commercial on. Wanna make out?" is not the mantra for inspiring cosmic sexual union. Many couples can dramatically shift out of old sexual holding patterns by completely revamping their bedroom. And you do not need to have a partner to create a sacred sleep chamber. Single ladies will also find that by creating a sacred sleep chamber, they too can open their sensual energy, freeing it for a new relationship or life project.

In general, these pointers will help you create an atmosphere that begs for sensual ritual:

- Keep the room light and airy. Open windows as much as the seasons allow.
- Keep the temperature mild and pleasant. Ayurveda recommends avoiding overheating or overcooling the room. Make sure your

body feels comfortable. Sometimes just feeling cold is enough to put out the sensual Fire.

- Get rid of the clutter. There should be nothing in the bedroom that reminds you of work. Move the stacks of papers you need to file at the office out of this sacred, sensual sleep chamber. Take the spare change and those piles of mail off the top of your dresser (go do it now, you know you have a stack like that!)
- Bring in harmony by keeping the room clean, beautifully painted, and orderly.
- The room should be private.
- There should be no machines or technologies in the room. Things that buzz kill the buzz. If you need to have an alarm clock, try finding one without bright lights and buzzing or ticking sounds.
- Decorations can reflect peaceful and romantic scenes.
- Create some boundaries on your eLife. Life changes when we make the adult decision to turn off our electronic devices after 9:00 PM. Seriously, the iPhone may be one sexy technological baby, but your significant other is yummier. Put it down. Please.
- The room should smell good but not too heavy. Avoid heavy incenses. Use fresh, romantic scents such as ylang ylang, vanilla, jasmine, and rose.
- The bed should be comfortable and not sag in the middle. Choose sheets that are made of natural, organic fibers.

Ayurvedic Techniques for Maximizing Sexual Vitality

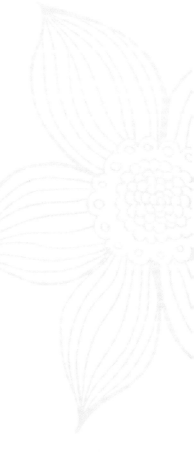

- Avoid sex within an hour of food.
- Remember, the ancient texts say the best way to build virility is by making love to someone who loves you. Sex with a partner that adores you boosts health and well-being more than any other technique.

- Well-digested food nourishes all of your tissues—the lymph, blood, muscle, fat, bone, marrow, and sexual fluids. When you take care of your digestion, you take care of your sexual essence. This essence, when used in harmony with nature, produces ojas—the foundation of your immunity and creativity. In other words, the food you eat has a direct effect on maximizing sexual vitality and overall energy levels.

- Don't overindulge. Ayurveda holds that too much sex may weaken your creativity.

- Approach sex as meditation. When sex is consecrated as a deep love ritual and made into a meditation, Ayurveda says that it can actually build our immunity and psycho-emotional strength. Making love with an attitude of complete surrender, with no fear or reservation, will boost trust and, in turn, build sexual health.

- Enjoying sex at night will be less energetically draining than sex during the day.

- Avoid having sex while menstruating (especially the first, heavier days).

- Making love during the full moon boosts sexual vitality, unless you are menstruating.

- After sex, urinate to get rid of any excess vata. A warm bath or shower is also good for relaxing after sex. Have a cup of warm milk. (See page 247 for postcoital tonics.)

- Don't use sex as a temporary stress reliever or painkiller. Use sex as a celebration of connection.

- Get out of the intolerable roles you play in your life. Ayurveda understands that if a woman feels unfulfilled in her life, or if she is performing a role she is in conflict with (i.e., being submissive to a husband when she doesn't want to be), her body will reflect this in the form of disease. Feeling that you are performing an intolerable role can create rigidity in the body, manifesting as stiffness (rheumatoid arthritis, for example) and dryness in your sexual and creative juices.

- Do not, I repeat, do *not* have sex that does not deeply satisfy you. If you are single, self-pleasuring is way healthier than unfulfilling and loveless sex.

Start Now: Meditation: Reclaiming Your Sexual Prana

Have the intention, over the course of a week, to remember and write down all of your sexual partners (any type of sex counts). When you feel that the list is complete, take some time to meditate. When you feel calm, go back through the list, person by person. Visualize them sitting in front of you. Actively begin to "call back" your own energy. As you inhale, see these unseen tubes of light returning to your womb and leaving the body of your past partner. As you exhale, offer back any unseen energetic connection that you may be holding with them. As you do this meditation, unprocessed emotion may arise. Simply let the emotions flow as you restore and reclaim your energetic sexual health. End the meditation by placing one hand on your womb and one hand on your heart. Hold compassion for yourself as you sense this reclaiming of your lost sexual energy.

You may need to do this slowly, one person at a time. By no means do you need to process the energy of all sexual partners in one session. Take your time. Observe celibacy while you are doing this process.

• • Essential Ideas • •

- Balanced sexual nutrition is just as important as food and sleep.
- Pleasure-power, or kama shakti, is the ability to perceive the sensual beauty that is always present. Tuning our five senses to the beauty of the present moment makes us feel like sexy creatures.
- Traditionally, women's sexuality has been taboo. Anything taboo results in feelings of shame.

- "Calling back" your sexual energy can be a powerful process for healing the past and making space for more love and pleasure-power in your life.

Putting Ayurveda to Work

- One of the best ways to experience an immediate surge in your pleasure-power is to meditate on the five senses. This week, give each of the five senses one full day of your attention. Every few hours during your day, stop and breathe. Remember the sense you are working with (seeing, hearing, tasting, touching, or smelling), and let that sensory capacity be the object of your meditation. What subtle colors, patterns, sounds, smells, or sensations emerge when you get quiet?
- Pick an afternoon or evening next week to practice the Meditation for Reclaiming Your Sexual Prana. Spend this week writing down past partners to prepare. On the night of your meditation practice, don't rush. Light candles. Let any emotions that may arise as a result of the practice flow through you.
- If you are in a relationship, share some of these ideas and practices with your beloved. It can be really fun to explore the five senses with a partner.

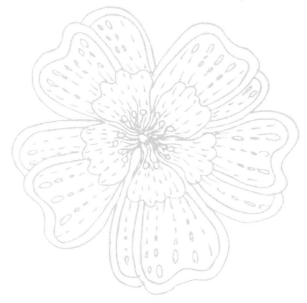

14

Tantra and Conscious Sex

First, let's dispel a couple myths. Tantra is not about sex, sex, and more sex, as long as possible and as many hours of the day. It is not ancient porn, nor is it an old-school manual for gettin' our groove on. Rather, it is a complex, highly refined, broad system for building energy and power in the worldly and the spiritual realms, weaving the two together for success in both. Think of it as the most complex, comprehensive, all-inclusive spiritual system ever developed. The word *Tantra* is from the Sanskrit *tan*, meaning "extension" or "expansion" and *tra*, meaning "to liberate" or "to release." So Tantra is about expanding our awareness to free ourselves and merge with the Divine. In other words, it can be defined as anything that asks us to stretch beyond our boundaries, to get out of our comfort zone, and to overcome the obstacles that keep us from deep fulfillment in all areas of our lives.

Sounds pretty amazing without needing to include sex!

Tantra offers us a methodology for living the most sublime, energy-filled, spiritually connected life possible. It includes a seemingly endless array of methods and knowledge for completing this sublime goal—Ayurveda, hatha yoga, astrology, gemology, herbology, architecture, interior decorating, dance, mantra, meditation, breath work, and yes, even sex. According to Tantra, both worldly and spiritual practices can contribute to us living the most energy-filled, healthy, happy life possible because the sacred and the worldly are one.

Tantra, like Ayurveda (which is a part of Tantra), does give some really great advice on how to get the most joy and power out of sexuality, but it also gives advice on how to decorate a room, make an herbal formula, raise a child, conduct business, work with the

> "She devours the world. She is called Kama (Desire). She gives with one hand and takes with the other. She is full of intelligence and strength. She is ever moving and difficult to suppress. She is a form of fire and we offer her oblations. "
>
> —*Atharva Veda* (author's translation)

breath and the body, as well as calculate the positioning of the planets and stars when we were born. Tantra's ultimate goal is the experience of spiritual enlightenment through total integration in the worldly realm.

So, sorry, sex-crazed kittens; if the book of Tantra were a mile high, the sexy parts would only reach a few feet into the air. In fact, the Kama Sutra itself was written by, ahem, men. And while I love men to death, I certainly would rather hear about the potency of my flowering lotus from Aunt Bessy than Uncle Bill.

Conscious Sex

In Sanskrit, there is a term for the evocative pleasure and love that arises between romantic partners: *sringara rasa*. Think of the first or best time you were in love. During this moment, all you could think of was that person. They could do no wrong. You may have even felt that the object of your affection was like a god or goddess. Your love and infatuation caused you to see only the best qualities in that person. You felt excited. But with time, that in-love feeling can wane.

The ancient Vedas taught that this love could get deeper and deeper, and in fact last a whole lifetime. Sadly, many times this initial love tends to weaken in people, and old patterns and reactions become the new template from which relationships function. Tantra teaches us how, through devotion, meditation, and an awareness of energy, to awaken a maturation of love and sexuality that transcends the initial falling in love. The practices in this chapter, and in this book, will help you cultivate sexuality and a zest for life that is enduring and independent of an outside lover.

Start Now: Wild Red Goddess

As the *Chakra Sambhara Tantra* suggested, "Visualize yourself as an erotic, red goddess, symbol of dedication and passion. Three eyes blazing with passion, your tongue is lustful with the purifying power of your inner fire. You are a naked goddess, with disheveled hair; symbolizing freedom from the bonds of delusion. You are intuition—a reminder that everything must pass. Blazing like fire, you express your wisdom essence, in embracing your lover without restraint."[1]

Shiva Rea describes sringara rasa as the archetypal union of male and female, sun and moon, stillness and dynamic movement, inhalation and exhalation. "It is a cultivation of the heart and sensuality . . . that helps us feel and generate loving energy toward ourselves, others, and ultimately the Divine . . . Instead of simply breathing, drink in the breath and allow it to travel from the base of the spine to the heart or to the crown of the head."[2]

We can use many methods—breath, yoga asana, development of the senses, and even sex, to tap into the heart's sensuality. Sex is a particularly ripe act for transforming our consciousness, due to the sensorial power of the experience itself. We can use sex as an unconscious, semiconscious, or fully conscious, consecrated act. In the conscious, sacred-sex approach, we use sex as a portal into Divinity. How? Well, many texts and respected teachers say the same thing—we must view our partner and the sexual act as Divine. We experience our partner, in our mind and heart, as the Divine manifestation of God or Goddess.

Practically, we can think about it as Tom Kenyon does in his book *The Magdalen Manuscripts*. Jesus (the divine masculine), he says, adored his woman (Mary Magdalen, the divine feminine) absolutely and completely. In turn, Mary trusted her man implicitly, without reserve, and from that trust she surrendered to him endlessly. Through this dyad of loving exchange, both Mary Magdalen and Christ were able to supercharge their capacity to embody universal power and love. Both men and women can hold these sacred roles for one another, as needed.[3]

Sex becomes sacred when we set aside purely personal goals of sensory pleasure. Conscious sex focuses on being present with and pleasing our beloved. Does this mean we should not communicate our needs, fantasies, and other sexual expressions? No, because if your partner is primarily concerned with pleasing you as a goddess, and you are primarily concerned with pleasing your partner as the Divine as well, then a clear line of communication on what each partner wants and desires begins to open up. If both partners want nothing more than to give love and pleasure to the other, then sex can open us into transpersonal ecstasy.

Sex becomes sacred when there is a merging. In harmonious, ecstasy-rendering sacred sex, there is a fusion of the partners' energy bodies. This fusion creates, for a moment in time, one body. If we are tuned in to our sensations without them overwhelming us, and we can keep a quiet mind, we can sense this Body of One.

The Kama Sutra likens the act of conscious sex to holding fire in one hand and water in the other. We want to keep the fire of our sensations and passions bright. But if the fire starts to get out of hand, and we get closer to climaxing, we can pour a little water on the act by coming back into our deep breath and a calm mind. We also don't want sex to become too "watery" or dull. The balance between fire and water is imperative to long-lasting sex that transcends short-lived orgasms. And whereas normal, biological, less-than-conscious sex is a steep mountain with a little tiny peak of brief ecstasy at the top, conscious sex is a broad plateau of sensation and experience that slowly rises and rises, offering more and more layers of satisfaction for both partners.

Start Now: Sacred Sex Ritual

Visualize your partner as Divine. Adore and trust him as the representation of all men, of the Divine Masculine made manifest. See his body as the sun. Feel that you can suck in the power of his rays, as you bathe him in the wet, white nectar of your moonlight. Make love together, deeply tuned to the excitement of physical pleasure, as well as the more subtle sensations and emotions that arise. Alternate periods of fast movement with periods of deep breaths and slowness—perhaps even silence and stillness. Visualize this creative, life-giving energy moving up through your collective body as one Divine Force.

The C Word

So, what if you aren't experiencing conscious sex? What if, in fact, you aren't really enjoying it at the moment? I can relate. I entered my late twenties in a whirlwind of dates with commitment-phobic men, several short-term boyfriends turned screamers and stalkers, as well as one man who left me because my breasts were "not big enough." I turned thirty emotionally drained, humbled, and ready to reassess my relationships. With the help of some powerful women guides, I decided that rather than diving headfirst into yet another prana-sucking relationship, I would try a stint of celibacy.

Now, before I go into my experiences with celibacy, let me first start by explaining a little bit about my family lineage. My grandaddy was nicknamed "Wild Bill," and my grandma, Mary Belle, was known for her striking good looks and Southern charm. In fact, the sexual nature of my family has become a kind of running joke, as we collectively reference our supreme fertility and sexual drive. The undercurrent in my family, and in our society at large, is that the ability to be sexually valued is equal to worthiness.

But I decided to stop the pattern and save my sanity. I underwent a period of celibacy, when I took my body off the market. I wanted to know who I was if I was not my sexuality. And it was not easy. I was one of those women whose sexual presence entered the room 10 minutes before she did. I found that, as I healed my sexual center, I noticed how much of my thought patterns, when engaged with the world, revolved around desirability. I sought out the eyes of attractive men. I noticed when men, and women for that matter, looked at me, and it felt good. But what if the day arrived when the world did not validate me? Who would I be?

Oftentimes, taking a break from sex can be a deeply soothing time. It is very hard to heal our heart if we are still engaged in sex. And there is no time limit. You may intuitively feel that you want a week off, a month off, or even several years off of sex. You may be happily married, and still need a break from engaging in sexual exchange. It is your right to do so, and it can be a time of deep healing, for you, the individual, as well as the collective feminine.

So, When Should I Sleep with Him (or Her)?

Maybe you've taken your time off, and now you're back in the game and think you're ready to get back out there . . . but you're not sure. Sorry, mama, there is no across-the-board correct answer to this. I know women who stayed "just friends" with a man for years and ended up divorced. I also know couples who got it on in the backseat of their car on the first date and are happily-ever-after types. The best advice regarding the when question is to look into one of the more delectable definitions of brahmacharya, which we discussed in regard to Ayurveda's three pillars. The more open-minded ancients weren't so concerned with *if* we had sex, but the intention behind it. They defined brahmacharya as "to walk with the Divine." If we are aligned with a higher power, whether through prayer or dance or meditation or any spiritual practice, then our body and clear mind will give an obvious indication about whether sex is a good idea or not.

The real-world Tantric mama knows better than to denounce her inherent sex-seeking nature. She enjoys her sexuality and has a "God made me this way" attitude about the whole matter. She may like showing off her great cleavage, but she does it from a place of celebration and comfort in her own sexy mama skin, and not because she is desperately seeking a man to gaze at her ta-tas. Similarly, she may decide to sleep with a man she has just met, but she does it from a grounded sense of their mutual intentions, his integrity, and a gut feeling that cannot be overlooked. This requires an extremely tight relationship to one's own self. And in my opinion, this can only come with sustained spiritual practice and lots of good ojas. When we have good ojas, we feel contained and content. When our immunity, both psychic and physical, is weak, we are more likely to make decisions based on lack and neediness, instead of strength and self-worth.

Celibacy Can Be Sexy

There's really nothing sexier than celibacy. It's a time of energetic gathering, when a woman can heal, detoxify (mentally and physically), and recharge her Spirit for her next creative expression. Choose a time to practice celibacy. It can be a few weeks or a few years. Both single and partnered women can practice it. Decide on the length of your celibacy. Make a contract that you will not break. Write it down. Use this time to clear out past negative experiences with partners or lovers. Forgive yourself and others. Hang out with people who support your decision. But most importantly, work with the practices in chapter 15 for deep sexual rejuvenation.

More often than not, the powerful goddess holds off on sex when she is entering a new relationship. In fact, most wise goddesses know that many men really like a woman who delights in allowing a man to court her for a nice long while. Indeed, most savvy mamas know that men, although they may not admit it, or even be aware of it, love the act of seeking her out. Why deprive them of this joy, ladies? And beyond their joy, the waiting allows you to experience the reality of the person in front of you, and you can make better decisions regarding your own desires and needs. That said, far be it from me to ask you to sign the "true love waits" petition I signed back in Vacation Bible School. There are no rules. Don't analyze. Stay grounded and make decisions from the silence of your soul.

The Twenty-One-Day Love Cloud

Oftentimes, we can't hear the voice of our soul, because we just aren't adept (yet!) at steeping ourselves in the kind of silence that informs our decisions. Then we start exchanging juicy fluids and reaching orgasmic heights with someone, running the risk of entering into a 21-Day Love Cloud. What is a Love Cloud? Dear ladies, it can occur at any time, and with even the most unoriginal of suitors. To understand this most pheromonal of phenomena, imagine the following scenario.

You decide to give in to (let's call him) Johnny's persistent attempts to take you out for coffee. Johnny seems about average: not particularly attractive nor especially funny, or even moderately successful, but nice and available. You go out a few times, and one steamy summer night things get a bit hot and heavy and you sleep with him. Within the orgasmic flood of several feel-good neurochemicals (dopamine and oxytocin), an odd feeling begins to take over. The next morning, you wake up to a torrent of thoughts, speculations, fears, hopes, and dreams. Johnny snoozes beside you, snoring, impervious to your mental undertakings.

You are officially in the Love Cloud, a 21-day period whereby a woman, flooded with the pleasure chemicals of the night before, begins to swing into full-mama protection mode. During this period, she can suddenly find herself inexplicably and unwaveringly attached to her new partner. And while this may not occur in every situation, most women will admit to having feelings of attachment to their sexual partners, no matter how much they try to convince themselves that it was just a casual roll in the hay.

Why is this? Biologically, we are designed to reap offspring, create community, and foster connection amongst our tribes. What is more, when we are in the Love Cloud, we begin to actually experience and see our fictitious-Johnny as a better version of the pre-sex Johnny we went for coffee with the week prior. Dr. Donatella Marazziti, a psychiatrist at the University of Pisa, studied twenty couples who self-described as "madly in love for less than six months." Now, granted they *were* Italian, but she found that when analyzing blood samples from the lovers, the serotonin levels of these new lovers were equivalent to the serotonin levels of obsessive-compulsive disorder patients.[4] Another leading researcher in the psychology of love, Ellen Berscheid, found that newly star-struck lovers often idealize their partner, magnifying their virtues and dismissing their flaws.[5] Psychologists suggest that we need these rose-tinted love goggles so that we will stay together and become attached.

From a Tantric perspective, it is super important that we acknowledge the innate wisdom of our bodies, while at the same time being aware of the certain power loss that can occur when we offer our sexual essence to a man who is not prepared to lovingly hold space for our natural need to nest, connect, and remain partnered. In other words, keep your rose-tinted glasses, ladies, but make sure to check in with your higher self before you get attached.

• • Essential Ideas • •

- Tantra is an ancient methodology for realizing the sublime potential of a human life: a limitless spiritual capacity within the body, a way to make the world Divine, and a pathway toward experiencing life as sacred.

- We can all have conscious sex by building our capacity to hold our focus on our partner, as well as our own internal sensations.
- Sometimes, a period of conscious celibacy is what we really need to recharge our batteries and get closer to who we are.
- Try not to overthink *when* is the right time for sex; stay focused on how you feel, making the decision soberly and with a conscious eye toward why you want to have sex, and not if you *should* be according to someone else's rules.

Putting Ayurveda to Work

- If you are in a relationship, consider reading this chapter to your partner. Ask him or her to practice conscious sex with you.
- Practice any of the meditations in this book *with* your beloved. Talk about your experiences together.
- If you are not in a relationship, feel thankful. You can use this time to practice sensual celibacy and really work the self-care techniques in this book!
- As a woman, it is important to enjoy the thrill of being in love, without being blinded by the Love Cloud. Have you ever been in a Love Cloud? Are you in one now? Take out your journal and write about what it would look like to be in love, while being simultaneously seated in your soul's wisdom.

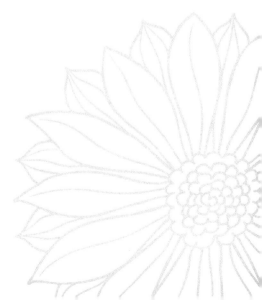

15

Cultivating Sexual Energy from Within

Within every woman lives a perfect goddess and an imperfect yet sacred harlot. You see, Tantra says that there is essentially no difference between our spiritual, kind, nurturing sides and our flirty, erotic, sex-loving sides. But if I'm being totally honest, this chapter is the one I spent the most time praying over. I felt that I was pushing against a cultural wall—that wall that says, "Be sexy, but don't talk about sex." In fact, I was tempted to cut a lot of the sexy stuff out of this book. But when I would talk to my female friends about the book and bring up sex, my friends clamored for more information—throwing questions at me, hungry to know more about how Ayurveda could help enhance their sexuality. It was clear that this was an important topic to write about, and it was important to share the wisdom that I've learned reignites our sexual aliveness.

And now it's time the cultural wall that separates women from their sacredness and their sexuality comes down. It's time we acknowledge that we are both spiritual and sexual creatures, and that it is okay. It's time we talk about our vibrant, pulsing, sexy selves without shame and denial. And it's time you learn how to build your sex power from within.

Tantra and Ayurveda both understand that sexuality can be a tool for spiritual transformation—or a tool for great pain and manipulation. We can see this understanding in the larger current cultural context whereby sexuality (mostly female, although not always) is misused to make money, sell products, and even enslave women. When we align with the ancient health practices around sexuality, we begin to experience an expansion on an energetic, physical, and emotional level that enables us to use our sexual power wisely and

191

from within. When we are tuned in to, and *turned on by*, our internal sexual aliveness, the likelihood that we will make decisions from an inner knowingness is dramatically augmented. In this way, we can better avoid the pain of harming others and ourselves through the misuse of sexual energy. And we can also say no when others may be overtly or covertly asking us to misuse this vital force. You are a spiritual and an erotic creature, and when both your inner virgin and your inner sex-goddess can find a home in you and flourish, the whole world will rejoice.

A Tantric View of a Woman's Energy

Within both Tantra and Ayurveda, a woman's energy (prana) is highly revered. When conserved and multiplied, sexual energy is seen as a powerful means to attaining physical rejuvenation and higher spiritual awakening. Within this worldview, you get to reach God while becoming sexier and healthier. Cool, huh? In ancient times, these practices were kept highly secret—they were the domain of queens and sacred temple priestesses. Luckily, human consciousness has evolved enough for these practices to now be made available to all of us.

Tantrics saw our organs—particularly our sexual organs—hormonal glands, and the nervous system as the physical leaping-off points for our evolution as human beings. When these organs are supercharged with our awareness, we have more energy and improved immunity, and a natural sense of contentment emerges. Working with sexual energy helps heal and restore these organs, boosting ojas and giving us more fuel for both our worldly ambitions and pleasure, as well as our spiritual goals.

The more loving energy we have flowing freely in these organs and systems, the more energy we have for life, and the sexier we feel. Men deplete this energy through excessive work, overthinking, and ejaculation. But women are different. Our ojas also gets depleted through overthinking and overworking—but not as much through orgasm, particularly not full-body orgasms. Our ojas gets greatly depleted through stress and unprocessed emotions, such as sadness, fear, anger, and shame. Another way our ojas gets depleted is when we menstruate (which is why we should rest then), but loving, full-body orgasms can actually build our energy. Furthermore, there are additional practices that conserve, transform, and transmute sexual energy. In this way, a woman (by herself or with a partner) can turn her raw sexual potency into a life force that can rebuild the power she loses from negative emotions and general life stressors.

Using Our Sexual Energy Wisely

Okay, so how do I build my sexual energy? First of all, work to process your negative emotions, whether through journaling, with a therapist, or by using other techniques you have come to rely on. Also, working to incorporate the practices in this book into your life builds sexual energy. Another way of building sexual vitality is to work with the energy-based meditation below.

The womb area (also known as the uterus, located in our lower pelvic area) is our feminine heart. It is the seat of our creative capacity, as well as where our ability to heal and rejuvenate our own body rests. The feminine womb is also a storehouse for much of our past pain, whether it is sexual trauma, abandonment, or other forms of abuse. Ironically, it is the center of pleasure and watery, creative power. Think of your womb as an oceanic force—dark and healing.

I have found that this area tends to be quite numb in many women, particularly if they have had any type of surgery on or removal of reproductive organs. This meditation is also extremely helpful for women who have lived through sexual abuse, as well as women who feel unfulfilled in their current sexual partnerships. Reclaiming this area involves bringing our attention to it, no matter how numb or painful it may feel. This meditation will help you feel at home in this part of yourself again. It is one of the single most powerful practices I have experienced as a woman.

Meditation for Healing and Building Sexual Energy

You can do this meditation sitting down, but I find it helpful to lie down with some support under my spine, such as a folded blanket or a bolster. Try working with this practice for at least 40 days, for 15–45 minutes daily.

Close your eyes and let your body relax and settle into its connection to the earth. Feel that you are in a nurturing, soothing place, and that you are fully safe to relax and let go. Notice, for a few minutes, the simple miracle of your breath. The inhale raises the navel center away from you, without you trying, and lowers the belly back onto you as you breathe out. Again, try not to try. Simply watch your belly as you become more and more relaxed.

Now, begin to smooth and even out the inhale and exhale. Take a few minutes to get the inhale and exhale as smooth and even as possible. The more relaxed you become, the subtler your breath becomes. Now, begin to remember love. Remember a time when you felt totally in love, totally safe, and totally nurtured. Take a few minutes to be in this memory of sweet love.

Slowly begin to become aware of where you feel love in your body. What is it like? Is it open or closed? Is it warm or cold? Expanded or contracted? Why does it feel good? Begin to let this love spread to your entire being. Rest for a moment in the love. Anytime you feel yourself coming into self-judgment, come back to the remembrance of love. Tell yourself, "My darling, you are seen; you are loved." Talk to your inner being like a little girl. Tell her everything is going to be okay. (We do this "little girl" talk because many of our painful patterns are stored from childhood.)

Begin to bring your attention into the space around your tailbone area, all the way around to your pubis and up to the space just below the navel. Blow your awareness up like a balloon at this area. Breathe in and feel your inhale inhabit your pelvic floor. Breathe out. Breathe in and feel your inhale inhabit your lower back. Breathe out. Breathe in and feel your inhale inhabit your right hipbone. Breathe out. Breathe in and feel your inhale inhabit your left hipbone. Breathe out. Now, breathe in and feel your inhale inhabit your entire pelvic bowl (sense this pelvic area that sits low and deep under your belly), the sacred sacrum, the holy place. Take a few minutes to let your awareness swirl around as love and energy in your sacred bowl. Search out any areas that may feel blocked.

When you find these spots, you can see them as blockages sitting on the vast creative capacity you hold in this area of your body, the seat of all rejuvenation and creation. Blockages also sit on the sweet pleasure that your pelvic bowl holds for you. Let your awareness stay in these spots, and keep breathing love, allowing your attention and focus to penetrate the dark corners of your feminine heart. Remember, energy follows focus. The more you can soften into love and send your focus to the stickiness, the greater the chance that the blockage can dissolve and resolve itself. Keep moving your awareness through the visualization and allowing the energy to open and disperse any blocks in your womb.

Finally, there may come a moment when the womb area is just so full of light and openness that you can abandon the technique and simply enjoy breathing into the new space you have created there. Now would be a good time to begin to chant a mantra into the energetic womb connection you have created. The mantra *som* [SOHM] is an excellent healing tonic for this area.

To come out of the meditation, simply deepen your breath while offering gratitude for the practice. Slowly begin to move your body and come back.

The Big O

It's pretty impossible to talk about sex without talking about orgasms. Energetically speaking, different orgasms create different kinds of energy. Clitoral and vaginal orgasms send energy down. Internal orgasms send energy in and up. The first type of orgasm can be exciting, a release, but also mildly depleting, especially if experienced without love. On the other hand, internal orgasms are not climax oriented but rejuvenation oriented, and travel through the internal organs, glands, and nervous system. Think of the clitoral or vaginal orgasm as Sex 101—a great thing to play around with and enjoy, but internal orgasms are definitely part of Advanced Sexuality.

To achieve an internal orgasm when engaging in sexual activity, such as lovemaking or masturbation, attempt to keep the orgasm from leaving you. In other words, concentrate on soaking in the sensations themselves. Stop seeking an eventual release. If climax and release happen that is fine, but try to direct the sensations upward and inside your body, into your ovaries, kidneys, and lower back area. Eventually, you may be able to direct the sensations higher into your navel, heart, throat, and head. If this happens, a woman can experience something beyond a clitoral or vaginal orgasm. It is as if the whole body is vibrating. In this type of internal orgasm, time seems to slow or stop and you merge with your partner—and even the entire Universe. Yes, that's possible, but it requires a great deal of love, trust, and most importantly, surrender. In this total-body orgasmic experience, energy isn't lost; it's gained.

In order to experience a full-body orgasmic experience, it's first vital that you train yourself to be sensitive to feeling energy and moving energy in your body. You can become better at this by practicing the meditations and energy work throughout this book, as well as the meditation we just did on page 194 (meditation for healing and building sexual energy). Remember, your energy follows your focus, so even if at first this feels a little foreign or is hard to feel, know that if you are focusing inside your body and moving your awareness through your body, you are moving energy! Eventually, you will be able to feel a clear channel of life force pulsing through you.

Once you feel more in tune with your own sensations and capacity to move sexual energy, you can practice full-body orgasms. Have your partner begin stimulating you in whatever sexual way feels good to you. You can also self-pleasure if you don't have a partner. Focus your attention on the sensations in your body. When you feel the sensations localized, for example, on your clitoris, begin to bring the focus upward to the ovaries. Keep concentrating your attention on this area until your whole lower back and belly form a uniform sensational field.

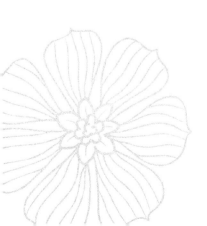

You may need to work on just bringing the sexual energy up to your navel for a few days or weeks. With time, you can begin to move the internal vibration and pleasure sensations up, up, and up—until they vibrate your whole belly, heart, throat, head, and even beyond your body. This takes time, practice, and is greatly augmented by the presence of a skilled partner who can hold the space for you to flower in.

Start Now: Tips for Practicing Full-Body Orgasm

When you are working to transmute and transform, don't worry if you get overly excited and come. It's all part of the practice. With time, you will get more skilled at working to move the energy up. You can also move this energy to parts of your body that need healing. And of course, you can also move this energy into your vagina and explode in a regular type of orgasm. It's all up to you. Internal, full-body orgasms are different for every woman (just as clitoral or vaginal orgasms can be different for different women). These orgasms often do not feel like a climax but more of a healing merging with all of Creation. I often find that when I am in the space of a full-body pleasure experience, there is no goal. And I often stop at the height of the experience and just rest in the healing energy of life, sex, and love.

In other words, there may not be an explosion, per se, but a heightened sense of awe and unity. I also find that the more I give myself to the totality of my body's pleasure capacity, the more I am totally turned on by life. A moonlit walk in spring can actually send my whole body into a semi-orgasmic state. I'm not vibrating, but I am smiling and feeling the subtle waves of pleasure pulse through my brain, my heart, my belly, and yes, my vagina.

Your Mind on Sex

It may not be obvious at first, but your vagina and your womb are not your most erotic sex organs. Your most erotic sex organ is your mind.

Jade Eggs

A wonderful physical practice for building pleasure-power is the ancient practice of working with jade eggs. An Eastern technique for keeping the muscles of the vagina and pelvis in general strong and flexible, jade eggs also increase the circulation of fluids in the vagina, help with incontinence, increase libido, and prime your lady parts for deeper sexual pleasure. Plus, isn't just the idea of putting an egg-shaped piece of jade into your sacred lotus enough to turn you on?

Working with jade eggs also offers us tremendous potential for bringing prana into our sexual center, strengthening a woman's energetic ability to feel sealed in, preventing her sexual energy from leaking out and downward. I have found this work to be incredibly powerful for building self-esteem and working to release many forms of trauma held in this sacred area of a woman's body.

How do I get this egg, you ask? Check my resources section for some good jade egg sources online. There are a multitude of sizes. I suggest buying 3–4 eggs of different sizes. The smaller the egg, the more work you will have to do to hold it in, so don't start too small. When you first buy your egg, make sure to boil it in water for about 20 minutes before using. You can also buy a jade egg with a tiny hole through the middle of it. You can run a string of dental floss through, tying the top end into a knot, to pull the egg out of your body if you are worried about it getting stuck.

Using your egg: There are many exercises you can do with your jade egg. Here is a simple one to get you started.

Lying on your back, bend your knees and place both feet on the floor. Begin by massaging your breasts. You can use a little sesame or coconut oil for added pleasure. This starts to activate hormone secretions throughout the body, making it easier for the egg to slide in. You can also self-stimulate the vagina as well. Then, if you need it, place some all-natural lubricant or sesame oil on the egg for added lubrication. When you feel aroused, bring the egg to the vaginal opening; slowly make circles with the fat end of the egg, massaging the vagina. As the vagina slowly begins to open, slip the egg inside (fat end upward). As you inhale, gently pull the pelvic muscles upward and draw the egg in and up. As you exhale, relax and lightly press the egg downward, toward the opening of your vagina. *Repeat*.

Try to feel a natural wavelike motion of energy in your body while using the egg. If you can do the waves on your breath, even better. The cervix will be the top part of the wave and the lower lips of the vagina will be the bottom. This is the part where you really strengthen the vagina and begin to have a lot more control over that part of your body. And while it is only a cursory benefit, this exercise makes sex so much more fun. For a male partner, your vaginal walls give him more sensations of massage and wavelike undulation. For you, the potential for longer, more powerful, and even multiple and full-body orgasms is increased.

The ancients understood that, especially for women, the realm of the mind was crucial in heightening the sensual experience. In order to supercharge your sex life, you've gotta start by training your mind. This is why the sexiest chapter of this book may not actually be this one, but the one on meditation. When we achieve a certain mastery over our thinking mind, we can direct this energy toward our sexual experience.

Here are some tips on improving your sexual experiences, no matter who they are with:

- **Cultivate your single-pointed focus:** One way of working with this idea is to concentrate on the sensual aspects of sex. When you are making love, tune in to all of your sensations and observations as if they were Divinity itself. For example, watch how your partner moves and shifts their body. How does she respond to your touch or gaze? What subtle changes happen in his skin color or smells? Look at his subtle gestures. Become a keen observer and responder to your beloved.

- **Do an emotional detox:** There is nothing that kills your sexy factor (and your orgasmic potential) in and out of the bedroom like emotional constipation. Mental and emotional blockage is at the root of our sexual dissatisfaction. Spending a few minutes really letting yourself feel your feelings (without repressing or resisting them) helps emotions unravel and "detox." Check out the "Putting Ayurveda to Work" section at the end of this chapter (page 201) for my personal emotional detox practice.

- **Invest in your self-esteem:** Another sexy killer is insecurity, self-doubt, and the "I'm not pretty (young, skinny, successful, etc.) enough" syndrome. There is a huge fallacy roaming our collective consciousness, exacerbated by porn culture, which says that women must look, move, and act a certain way during sex. Nothing could be farther from the truth. Sexiness comes not from dressing a certain way, having a certain grooming habit, or wearing certain lingerie. If you only work to attain a superficial sexuality, based in consumer culture, sexual insecurity will not go away. In fact, this false sexual drama drains and depletes sexual energy. Knowing your inherent worth and beauty builds sexual energy from inside. It is a recipe for irresistibility.

Beyond Orgasm

When we consider everything we've covered so far, we're already well on our way to moving past superficial sexuality, but we also need to move beyond the big O. We tend to think of orgasm as the end goal, and perhaps multiple orgasms as the realm of a few lucky women. But Tantra—and our true sexuality—is more than orgasm. Tantra is a practice that teaches you how to tune yourself—spiritually, energetically, and physically—to the beauty and pleasure of life. In this way, everything you encounter becomes an opportunity to merge with the Divine. Furthermore, through the practices of growing your own relationship to energy, like using meditation, deeper and deeper states of pleasure are reached—on your own. There is nothing wrong with clitoral or vaginal orgasms. Have them! But keep in mind that both Tantra and Ayurveda say there is an internal experience, called enlightenment, that makes an orgasm feel like a sneeze. So, practice the techniques in this chapter in conjunction with the soul-revealing techniques in chapter 12.

• • Essential Ideas • •

- A woman can be a spiritual, kind, mothering being and at the same time a sweaty, erotic, sex-loving being. They are both equal and perfect expressions of her Divinity.
- Your sexual energy should be highly revered. It is the potential you have for worldly and spiritual awakening.
- Your sexual energy can be used for healing the physical and emotional body. It can also be reinvested into creative pursuits. Use it lovingly and wisely!

Putting Ayurveda to Work

- Practice the meditation on page 194 before working with orgasm practices in sex. This will clear the womb and sexual organs of stagnant energy, and prepare you to be more sensitive to the energy of sex. This meditation will also help boost your focusing power for heightened sexual experiences.

- Buy your jade eggs this week! Get our your journal and write down any interesting sensations, revelations, or emotional experiences that may arise.

- Here's my personal emotional detox practice for you to try this week at home: Spend a few minutes feeling these four emotions: anger, sadness, fear, and guilt or shame. Finish this sentence on paper or aloud: "I am angry that _____." Repeat this as many times as needed to express all the ways you are angry. Start each sentence with "I am angry that . . ." to avoid analyzing. Really let yourself *feel* the emotion. Move into sadness and continue until all the sadness has left your body. Do the same thing with fear and guilt. Finish with a powerful, positive statement about yourself, your body, and your life. Repeat the powerful, positive statement 10 times—or until you really believe it!

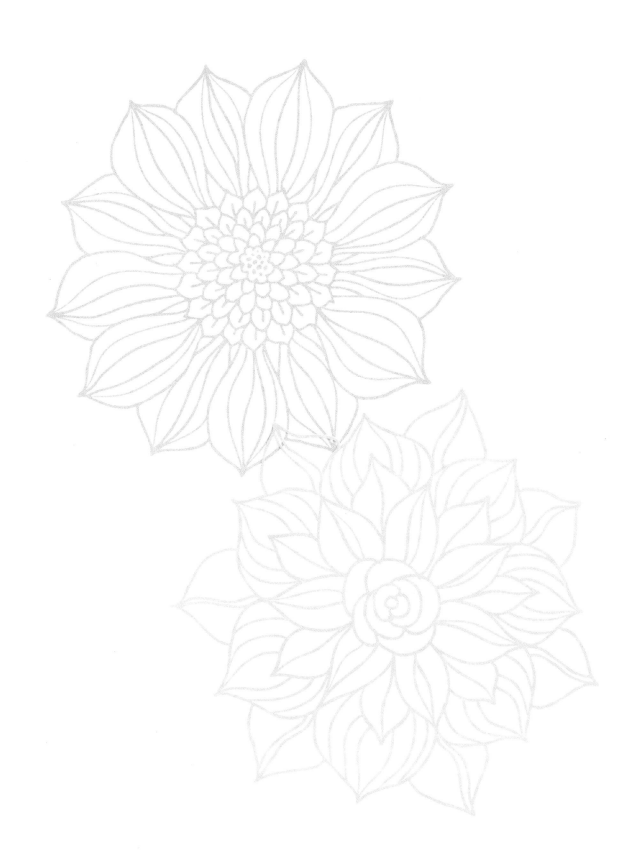

16

The Power of Your Womb

There is nothing sexier than self-esteem. And there is nothing that builds self-esteem more than walking courageously into the depths of our own experiences and feelings. One of the most enlightening and surprising realizations I came to with Ayurveda and my own journey toward self-esteem and sexuality is how the seat of female power lies in the womb—the dark, fleshy home of our creative energies. What I learned is that, in this sacred female womb, we create. Our creation makes babies, births social activism projects, produces art, bakes bread, and starts businesses.

I also learned that the womb is the seat of our destructive powers. In this sacred female womb, we bleed, feel pain, and slough off a layer of who we are each month. This destruction is necessary for creating anew.

The female womb is also the seat of our deepest emotional mystery, pulling us down and out each month, asking us to deeply feel the truth of what we didn't process the month prior. This center is the home of our unconscious lust, and in it dwells our secret desires, hopes, and longings. It's why, at various times of the month, our sensitivity can be more intense—when we might feel our most vulnerable both physically and emotionally. If this center is blocked or numb, we may feel disconnected from our creativity and sexuality. When this center is undernourished and unloved, we may experience a disconnection from, or even a hatred for, our menstrual cycle or our menopausal process.

By honoring your natural female cycles, you can begin to align yourself with the greater cycles of the moon, tides, and seasons. Through honoring the pain that may be present in the womb at various times of the month or of your life, you can build a relationship to all aspects of who you are. This relationship to the womb asks us to not avoid the pain by running toward quick external fixes that block the flow of sensations and experiences. In my own experience, and my own body, I am astounded at how healing my relationship to my creative center has enabled me to be the full spectrum of who I am as a woman—the lovable, wise woman and the wounded creature. In this, I am integrated and I become whole.

Sexiness is an expression that naturally emerges from a woman who walks in this wholeness. This wholeness makes room for the pains of loss, childbirth, and unmet expectations. This wholeness also makes room for the pleasures of orgasm, fulfilled longings, and grace. Let your womb, and your menstrual experience, be a time of celebration and healing, and you will be one undeniably sexy creature—of this I am certain.

Our Menstrual Experience— A Curse or a Cure?

You are a living miracle once a month. Canakya, the ancient Indian philosopher, once said, "Bronze gets cleaned with acid. River gets cleaned by its own forceful flow, and a woman is purified with menstruation."[1] So even though we are purified during this time, many of us experience our menstrual cycle as a painful and inconvenient mess. Painful menstrual experiences are not normal. Bloating and cramping are not normal. Excess bleeding and infertility are not normal. For the modern woman, these symptoms may be *common*, but they are not normal. In fact, our periods are actually connected with our juicy, life-giving prana. If we have scanty periods, our prana is depleted. If we have heavy periods, or stagnation, our channels for healthy prana are blocked.

Many Ayurvedic physicians from India who visit the West are astounded by the major imbalance we Western women are experiencing in our menstrual cycles. Difficult and painful PMS and menopause are largely a Western experience. Why? Because we have dishonored the cycle of nature. In the East, the menstrual cycle is highly revered as the sacred feminine that is synced to the cosmos by way of the moon. It is well known that women require lots of extra energy to have an effective bleeding and cleansing process, and traditionally, women went into red tents to rest and enjoy their solitude or be with other women. These rituals created important bonding experiences with other women. Feeling supported by a tribe of women during her "dark days" of bleeding was an essential part of woman's health.

But you and your friends don't need a red tent. You can start to honor your sacred time as a cleanse and cycle of rejuvenation by working to stabilize your menstrual cycle. Consider scientist Margie Profet, who won a MacArthur Foundation genius grant for her work in fertility and menstruation. Her theory, which is supported by Ayurveda, is that the menstrual cycle has evolved as a way of nourishing and replenishing the feminine reproductive organs. The rich, immune-boosting blood washes through the body in a way that no other type of blood can. It literally cleanses the uterus, cervix, and vagina with powerful antibacterial and antiviral agents.[2]

This is why it is so crucial to not ignore your periods any longer. Ayurveda states that menstrual difficulties can usually be traced back to a number of root causes. Consider these questions to figure out your personal history with menstruation and start from a place of knowledge:

- Were your natural urges for sexual expression suppressed?
- Did you feel supported in your transition into womanhood, or was it a time of embarrassment and suppression?
- Were you sexually abused, or did you experience trauma around sexuality? Did you have excessive amounts of sex?
- Did you overexercise as a young woman? Do you now?
- Was your diet composed of whole foods like vegetables, fruits, and grains? Or was it heavy on meats, dairy, and processed foods? Did you eat junk food? Were you overweight? Did you have an eating disorder?

These are all questions to reflect upon when looking at the root causes of menstrual difficulty.

The Pull of the Moon

PMS has become the victim of many a joke in our modern, patriarchal world. Seen by our culture as an emotionally volatile state when women become hormonally hysterical, overly sensitive, and uncontrollably hungry for ice cream, it is no wonder that most women feel ashamed of their menstrual cycle. From Eve's apple onward, our culture has done much to repress feminine power. Our blood and menstrual cycles were considered dirty and evil. Women were not allowed in sacred spaces during our menstrual flow. And even today, women carry a collective unconscious shame-burden around their female blood-based reality.

In general, works such as *Malleus Maleficarum* (which translates to "witch's hammer") and the behavior of the Roman Catholic Church during the 1400s fostered a belief that women were untrustworthy, deviant, and the cause for the demise of man. Women who knew a lot about delivering babies were killed off; chicks who understood how plants could be used for healing were burned at the stake. Heck, women who played with dogs and cats too much were considered witches! Men took over all tasks related to caring for women's health, and in this shift toward the masculinization of women's health, we began to lose our direct connection to the magic and power of our own menstrual flow.

Within this historical environment of shamed womanhood, it is no wonder that statistics show that at least 85 percent of American women experience at least one symptom of PMS every month.[3] It is also easier to push away the unpleasant darkness that it can bring up, rather than feel the feelings. Indeed, my own travels across the country talking to women confirm that women are suffering, especially in regard to their reproductive health. Their bodies are speaking to them very clearly in the form of pain, tenderness, anxiety, depression, and even deeper imbalances. And the message is an unequivocal: "Hey, mama, something is out of whack." We are experiencing a strong denial of our pain body.

What Is a Pain Body?

Author and spiritualist Eckart Tolle defines pain body as "the remnants of pain left behind by every strong negative emotion that is not fully faced, accepted, and then let go of." When we aren't able to fully process our emotional experiences, this pain forms an "energy field that lives in the very cells of your body."[4] If you refuse to take time out to feel it, your pain body begins to speak louder and louder. And not only is our body a storehouse of these past experiences, but it is also a storehouse for things that have happened to our mothers, sisters, grandmothers, and the collective feminine. These gorgeous bodies allow us to experience both the pleasure and bliss of being a human being, as well as all the pain, trauma, and negativity that our emotional investments and past experiences have held on to over years and lifetimes.

In ancient times, women usually bled together. Their periods aligned with the pulls of the moon. We went into special huts, far from the fires of our kitchens and the needs of our families. Grandmas and older children stayed with the babies, as the collective community acknowledged the importance of this collective female downtime. In this safe space, we bled and told stories and prayed and meditated. We got together, in solitude, because our power was so great that whatever we focused on became supercharged. This is a testament not to the inherent dirtiness or pain of our time of the month, but to the wild, raw power of the event itself.

Today, because we lack a container for the power of our lunar days, we suffer. We force our hemorrhaging bodies out into the bright lights of the office cubicle. We sit through traffic, push ourselves to spin class, take care of the kids, and continue with the same manic rhythms that we impose on ourselves during the other weeks of the month. This brings us not only out of sync with Nature's call for us to slow down and rest, but also prevents us from tapping into the very power of our lunar cycle in which we deeply feel. Simply stated, our menstrual cycle can be a time in which we can let go of any toxic emotions or holding patterns that we accumulated the month before. If we do not allow ourselves the necessary time and space for this to be felt as a visceral, emotional, and spiritual experience, we dishonor the very power that we are, perhaps, longing for all month long. Not only can we slow down during our menstrual cycle, but we should also take exquisite care of ourselves.

Let's look at a breakdown of the female lunar, or menstrual, cycle and its gifts:

- **Week One—The Scarlet Flow:** Day one of your lunar cycle begins when you start to bleed. Even within hours of starting your flow, your estrogen levels slowly begin to rise. Many women feel a sense of ease and flow as the estrogen returns and the heaviness or PMS subsides. The gift of this flow? That we can now release fully; enjoy the downward pull. This is a great time to feel any emotions that have been repressed or unnoticed during the busy weeks before. It is also the time to stop the momentum of creation. Rest. Give yourself permission to not be social.

- **Week Two—The Energy of Estrogen:** The second week of your cycle usually feels really good. You have undergone a natural form of bloodletting in week one, but now, during this time in your cycle, estrogen steadily builds. The gift of this week? Increased estrogen causes a spike in serotonin, the feel-good chemical associated with vitality and excitement about life. The second week of our lunar cycle is a great time to have important conversations, inspire others, celebrate, or launch a proposal.

- **Around Week Three—Fertility and Animal Magnetism:** Women typically ovulate (release an egg from the ovaries) around days 12–16 of their cycle. The gift of this part of the cycle? You can get pregnant (if that's your desire), and you experience heightened sensuality and strong magnetism. Studies even show that men find the same women's faces and voices significantly more beautiful during their ovulatory period.

- **Around Week Four—The Quiet, Intuitive Moon:** After ovulation, estrogen and testosterone begin to fall as progesterone levels rise. If the menstrual cycle is the moon, high estrogen is the full moon, and high progesterone is the new moon. When progesterone is high, you may experience some of the classic PMS and "I feel crazy" symptoms. You aren't crazy—your body is asking you to not engage with the world as much. These feelings, especially the emotional ones, arise when we go against our natural moon (which is asking us to turn inward) and try to behave as we were during our high estrogen cycle. Ancient shamanic traditions understood the new moon as the peak of intuition, deep insight and psychic capacities. Give yourself fully to your inner practices of meditation and self-inquiry. It's natural to feel less social and more inward during this phase of your cycle.

Super self-care is the principle way a woman can use her menstrual cycle for tuning in to her Higher Self. I suggest marking your calendar for the days that you know you will be most sensitive and powerful in regard to your connection to your own monthly moon energies. During your moon time (bleeding days), slow down as much as possible. If you are lucky enough to create your own work schedule, take 2–3 days off completely to restore and renew. Light candles. Meditate. Talk to your best friends.

Start Now: Breathe into Your Roots

To expand into our sexual fullness and heal energetic balances, we must first create an open, wide base in which energy can move. Many of the women I work with have a lack of prana moving in their pelvic bowl. How alive do you feel at your roots? If you close your eyes, what does it feel like "down there"? Assess the situation with love, and then practice this meditation for increasing prana in your sacred pelvic bowl.

Close your eyes and sit comfortably with the spine straight, or lie down. Feel your whole body begin to relax. Take a few moments to watch your breath; let it become even, smooth, and full. As you feel your body beginning to relax, take your awareness down into your pelvic root and bowl. Without judgment, look around down there with your inner felt-sense. Are there spots that feel alive, vibrating and full of light? Are there spots that are tense, scary, dark, or numb?

Take a few moments to breathe your presence into the realms that feel stuck, numb, or emotionally or physically painful. Feel that you can access energy from outside of the body as you inhale, and on the exhale, direct it into the stuckness, allowing it to dissolve. Do this for 5–10 minutes. As you begin to notice energetic shifts, there may be emotional releases that accompany this meditation. Try your best not to judge the release, but to let it unravel. Come back to your practice, and back to your breath. After 10 minutes, begin to visualize a downward-facing dark-blue triangle, its apex pointing downward toward earth at your tailbone, and the base as wide as your hips. When you feel your body breathing in, sense your awareness and energy moving through the dark-blue triangle and down to the tip, concentrating there. As you feel your body exhale, sense any holding, tension, toxins, or unwanted emotion leaving through the tip and moving down into the earth. Repeat this visualization and movement of energy 8–12 times.

Also, let all the excretions and fluids and pains flow freely. This is especially true of emotions and tears. Judith Orloff, in her book *Emotional Freedom*, states:

Tears are your body's release valve for stress, sadness, grief, anxiety, and frustration. . . . Like the ocean, tears are salt water. Protectively they lubricate your eyes, remove irritants, reduce stress hormones, and they contain antibodies that fight pathogenic microbes. Our bodies produce three kinds of tears: reflex, continuous, and emotional.

Each kind has different healing roles. . . . Typically, after crying, our breathing, and heart rate decrease, and we enter into a calmer biological and emotional state. Emotional tears have special health benefits.[5]

No matter what you're feeling, let yourself feel it. Indulge the tears if you need. Find and revel in the support you want. Honor your cycle through being aware of and letting yourself feel what arises.

Other Ways to Honor the Lunar Cycle

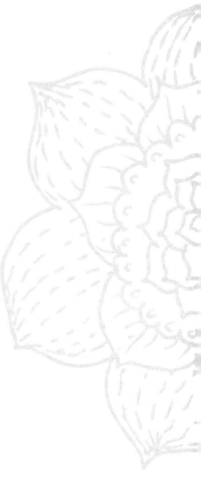

- **Take a time-out from technology.** Technology, in all of its elegance and efficiency, is different from goddess energy, which is inherently connected to the natural world. During your lunar cycle, it's a good idea to spend more time in nature, practicing silence, and less time on Facebook.

- **Go au naturel.** Think about what chemicals you put in to your sacred body. Avoid all tampons that hold chemical residues or dyed cotton. Buy a good natural brand (see the resources section). Switch to pads, when you can, as it allows the lunar waters to flow more freely.

- **Feed the earth your lunar waters.** A powerful practice for feeling connected to Mother Earth is to feed her your blood. Use a menstrual sponge or a moon cup (see resources page 276) to gather your blood. Simply use this blood to water your houseplants, or if you prefer, your garden outside. Blood is so rich with life force and nutrients. Why let it go down the drain when you could feed another being? When I do this, my plants become robust with life power!

- **Get more rest.** Make sleeping through the night, for 7–9 hours, a big priority. Often, just getting enough sleep can dramatically alter your periods. This should be a time of rest.

- **Stop taking in chemicals.** Avoid antibiotics, pesticides, and hormonal additives in foods, and chemical cleaning agents that contain harmful substances which can alter your menstrual cycle.

- **Think twice before pill popping.** There is nothing wrong with grabbing an aspirin in times of need, but many women pop everything from Midol to Prozac as a way to keep up the rat-race pace instead of allowing themselves to rest. Mild aches and pains are just your body's natural warning system, asking you to renew yourself. Usually, one day off and a good night's sleep can cure simple imbalances. Problems begin when these imbalances accumulate over months and years of not heeding the wisdom of our lunar cycle.

- **If you are on the pill, reconsider.** I know that this is not a popular option, especially for modern career-minded women, but here is the thing—menstrual blood helps cleanse the organs and kill off any foreign invaders (and by the way, men's sperm is rife with bacterial friends). With every period, you literally clean out any foreign bodies in your holy womb. This is probably why many of us actually feel "cleansed" from a past lover or life's experience after a good menstrual cycle. If you are taking a pill that alters or even eliminates this natural cycle, you may be missing out on one of the best immune-boosting, life-giving processes in your life. There are many other reasons why we may want to reconsider taking hormones, such as estrogen and progesterone. New and emerging scientific evidence actually shows a clear link between taking oral contraceptives and depression, nausea, headaches, and loss of libido. In 2005, the World Health Organization's cancer research group listed the pill as "carcinogenic to humans."[6]

- **Cook for yourself every day.** It sounds simple, but this truly is the number one way to change all aspects of your health.

- **Ditch toxic foods.** Avoid processed or nonorganic meats, alcohol, nonorganic and processed dairy, processed forms of sugar, sodas, and other nonorganic forms of caffeine.

- **Get off the bean.** The chemical constituents of coffee beans have a particular harmful effect on female reproductive tissue. Coffee is also usually sprayed with harmful estrogen-mimicking chemicals. If you are truly addicted to coffee, at least make sure that you are drinking an organic brand, and drink it with some milk or cream to reduce its acidic effects.[7]

- **Try a grounding meditation.** Visualize your legs and tail-bone as being powerfully rooted into the earth. Sense a strong, grounding presence that links your roots into the hot red lava at the center of the earth's core. Feel that the warmth and power of your womb is a mirror of the lava-power at the center of our planet. Visualize a downward pointing triangle at the base of the spine, pulling any toxic emotions, thoughts and old hurts, and anything you're holding on to out of you. A full version of this meditation is on page 157.

Balancing the Doshas to Balance Your Cycle

It takes some time to rebalance our systems, so while you are working to apply many of the Ayurvedic concepts of this book into your daily life, you may still have to deal with residual menstrual symptoms and PMS. Here are some ways to make the experience of menstruation a little more manageable, according to their doshic origin. And remember, rule number one prior or during your period: Act in accord with how you feel.

Vata Cycle

In general, drier, darker blood and scantier flows is indicative of more vata in the system. Vata periods also present with more clotting. Vata is also characterized by: nervousness, pain that is mobile or erratic or both, anxiety, spacey feeling, cramps, sparse or scanty periods (amenorrhea) that are often darker in color, insomnia, constipation, bloating, low back pain, and at the beginning or before a period, cravings for salty or savory foods.

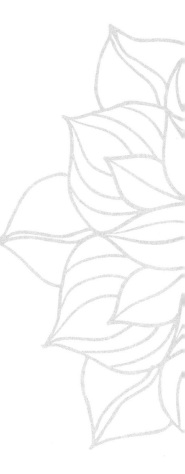

To deal with excess vata:

1. Think warm, wet, and grounding, in terms of food and lifestyle.
2. Rest, do some light, slow-moving yoga. Take a walk. Do not run. Allow yourself a few days off of any strenuous exercise while menstruating.
3. Massage the body in warm sesame oil.
4. Place 5 drops of nasya oil in each nostril, particularly if you are prone to headaches.
5. Eat sweet potatoes, squash, avocado, and Omega-3-rich fish.
6. Good herbs for vata-type PMS: ashwagandha, shatavari, turmeric, aloe vera, brahmi, nutmeg, triphala
7. Good teas for vata-type PMS: peppermint, rosehips, dried orange peel, cinnamon, clove, cardamom, ginger, and saffron in milk
8. Eat from the vata-reducing recipes on pages 236–242.

Pitta Cycle

Pitta periods tend to flow heavily the first few days, as the high heat brings a strong flow that tapers off. Some other pitta period issues are: crankiness, pain that is sharp and intense, irritability, criticism of self and others, anger, rage, acne, hot flashes, excess bleeding that is bright red in color and hot, burning, rash or inflammation, and cravings for sweet and spicy foods.

To deal with excess pitta

1. Think cooling, sweet, and calming, in terms of food and lifestyle.
2. Rest or do some light, slow-moving yoga or Tai Chi.
3. Avoid deadlines and competition.
4. Avoid caffeine, alcohol, and pungent (spicy) foods.
5. Massage your body with warm coconut oil.
6. Place 5 drops of nasya oil in each nostril, particularly if you are prone to headaches.
7. Eat bitter greens, asparagus, berries, coconuts, dates, spelt, oats, barley, and ghee.

8. Good herbs for pitta-type PMS: shatavari, vidari kanda, aloe vera, turmeric, licorice, brahmi, and manjistha

9. Good teas for pitta-type PMS: raspberry leaf, rose petal, fennel, lavender, ginger (fresh), saffron, nettles, and dandelion

10. Eat from the pitta-reducing recipes on pages 229–235.

Kapha Cycle

Kapha menstrual flows start slow and are moderate throughout. Kapha flows can feel heavy, and have mucus and moist, large clots. They also involve: thick blood that may have heavy clotting, whitish color or mucus, dull pain, water retention, depression, lethargy, emotionality, nausea, and swollen breasts, as well as cravings for heavy, sweet foods.

To deal with excess kapha

1. Think light and warming, in terms of food and lifestyle.

2. Do quicker-moving yoga. This will stimulate lymph and blood flow, as well as the flow of prana. Squats, lunges, and hip and groin openers are particularly helpful for dealing with an Aunt Flow that won't let go. Once your period starts, cease any strenuous exercise for at least the first few days.

3. Emphasize pungent and astringent tastes.

4. Massage the body in warm almond oil, or brush the body with a dry brush to move lymph.

5. Place 5 drops of nasya oil in each nostril, particularly if you are prone to headaches.

6. Eat bitter greens, asparagus, berries, coconuts, dates, spelt, oats, barley, and ghee.

7. Good herbs for kapha-type PMS: ashwagandha, manjistha, gokshura, vacha, ginger, and trikatu

8. Good teas for kapha-type PMS: rosehips, hawthorne berry, orange peel, ginger powder, lemon balm, hibiscus leaf, nettle, and fresh lemon juice

9. Eat from the kapha-reducing recipes on pages 224–228.

• • **Essential Ideas** • •

- Sexiness naturally emerges from a woman who has an energetic connection to the creative and destructive center of her womb. This connection is established through making room for the pleasure and pain that come from this female center.
- Both menstruation and menopause are times when women have access to more intuition. They are times when turning inward and stopping the momentum of giving to the outside world will result in more energy for higher pursuits.
- Understanding the relationship between your menstrual experience and the doshas can be a powerful tool for bringing hormonal balance. When our hormones are balanced, we naturally and effortlessly feel sexy.
- The pain body is the residue of past, undigested emotion. When we are unable to fully process our emotional experiences, this pain forms an energy field. A woman who is consistently living in her pain body has a hard time feeling sexy.

Putting Ayurveda to Work

- Practice the Breathe into Your Roots meditation on page 209 for at least a week or longer. Keep a daily log of your experiences. Notice how things change each day.
- Notice the deeper pain of PMS or menstruation. The time around our period can bring forth old emotion. This is a gift because it allows us to process the pain body. Here are some journaling ideas that might help you digest old feelings: "How have I abandoned myself this month? Where has my truth been suppressed? What emotions have I stuffed under the covers? How am I really feeling in my relationships? Am I sexually alive and satisfied?"

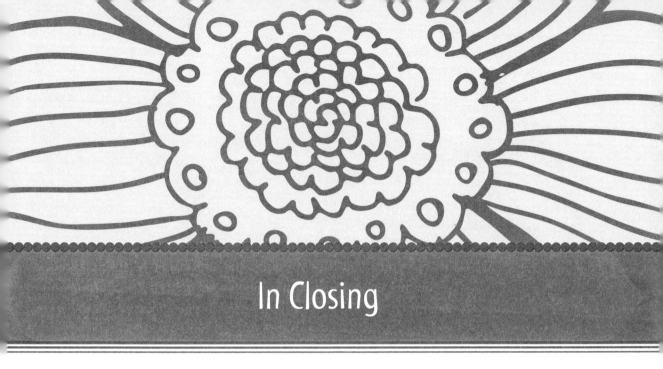

In Closing

Ayurveda is an offering: it is a gift from Mother Nature to us. And this book has been my offering in honor of Ayurveda: from my heart to yours. If Ayurveda and its ancient secrets does for you what it did for me, I know you are now on the path to being healthier, happier, and sexier than you ever imagined. And remember, you are not alone in your endeavors to live a more fulfilled, healthy, soul-driven life. In fact, you are connected to an unseen web of support.

This web is made up of women (and men), all over the world, who are waking up to the hidden wisdom traditions. It is woven with healers in forests attempting to preserve their sacred indigenous technologies. This web is softly strengthened by anyone who prays for someone else with an earnest heart. It is braided with the courage-strings of every woman who says "no more" to an abusive relationship. It is spun out of the collective inhales and exhales of millions of yoga practitioners, worldwide, who seek to calm their minds, even for the briefest of moments in the madness of modern living. It is knitted with the kindness of all beings who take care of sick children and dying elders. It is intertwined with women who, for the first time in many years, are removing the veil of shame that keeps them from admitting that they are living lives they don't fully want to live. This web is also lovingly crafted out of the Big Mama's strongest longing for you to awaken to yourself as spirit. And this web is getting stronger every day.

If there was one core Ayurvedic golden nugget I could slip into your pocket before this book finishes and we part ways, it is this: *You are intimately connected to everything.* The abiding spirit of Ayurveda shows us that there is an underlying natural order that holds and sustains all of us. We are made up of this infinite, all-pervading intelligence. When you make the commitment to living in greater harmony within yourself, you augment harmony for everyone and everything. You tap into limitlessness and become a walking "answered prayer." In this way, all of daily life becomes an expression of the fact that life is sacred.

Let the ancient wisdom of the Ayurvedic elders take root in your mind. Let that wisdom live in your heart as an unending, silent place that can guide you back to health and well-being. May your wellness be the fuel upon which you achieve your greatest life's purpose. And may the wellspring of your fulfillment inspire others to do the same.

In Love,

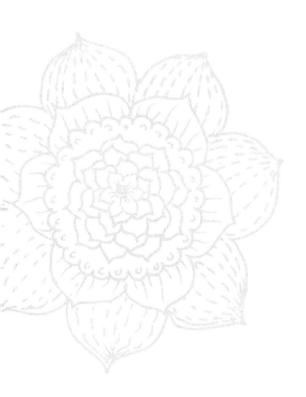

Acknowledgments

To the Sri Vidya and the Himalayan lineage. To my continual Divine Mama and your gentle sidekick, Jesus Christ-Consciousness—hopefully this book is in your service, my small step in bringing myself and the world back into sanity. Thank you for your fierce lessons and gentle arms. Beloved guru and friend Yogarupa Rod Stryker—I am grateful to be your *shishya*. Without your guidance (and your book), this book may never have been born.

For my mother, Vera Silcox, I chose you. I looked down from the heavens before I even had a body, and said to the gods, "Please, let me have that one, because she is an angel—a saucy angel." Thank you for birthing me, raising me, and letting me move back in with you to finish this book. For my father, Larry Silcox, for always telling me I was smart, and that he loved me. And for making me laugh.

For Wyatt, my brother, for being the only man who has ever bought me a bed, put my books on shelves and stuffed dollar bills into my socks. For Mary, my sister, my best friend, and my co-yogini on the path toward the Big Mama Love. Thanks for being the embodiment of so much of the Feminine Healer, to which this whole book is dedicated. You can cook. You can deliver a baby. You can spin vinyl records. You have a booty like a freight train and a heart after God. What could be better?

To Chrisandra Fox Walker, my pseudo-wife. For being my most insightful yogini sister. For your unending ability to pull the Holy Ash of Pure Truth out of the Beautiful Cow Shit of My Emotional Spins. Your presence on this planet reminds us that Love is Real, and that women are powerful because of their emotions. Thank you for embodying the weaving of samadhi into the real world. And for Robbie and Harry-hoo.

Deep, deep gratitude to Michael Rubin, for telling me the book had promise, despite his doubts about smelling like sesame oil. For your countless unpaid hours of editing. And for telling me, "Listen kid, the Dalai Lama himself could call you up and say, 'Hey, I wanna publish your book.' But you still have to write the book. So finish the book already." Michael, this book would not be in our hands right now if it weren't for you.

To my first editor, Margot Silk Forrest—you edited this book as if you were inside my brain and heart. For Ayurvedacharya Mary Thompson for your kindness, and your expert edits. For my amazing editors at Beyond Words, Emily Han and Gretchen Stelter. You guys "got it" from the very beginning, and challenged me every step along the way. Thank you for making this book-baby with me.

For Raghu Markus and Dr. Saraswati Markus for your kindness and willingness to give this project your love and attention. For Kelle Walsh, editor of *Yoga Journal Online*. Thanks for believing in the yoga and the writing. I can't tell you how much your support meant to me at such a vulnerable time in my life. For Richard Rosen, your time and your edits. For Martine Holston for being a business/cheerleader/ form-filler-outer, and midwife-editor to this book. To Barbara Gabriel for initiating me, and holding me, in the shamanic portals of the emotions. To Joe Barnett for letting me borrow your man cave in New Mexico where I wrote much of this book. To Jeff Stegman for your dharma on the planet, and for teaching me surrender. To Cole Nelson and Stevie Long at Spafit for being cheerleaders and amazing trainers. To Sherri Jessee for all your support and making me feel so beautiful.

To Sianna Sherman, Seane Corn, Dr. Claudia Welch, and Trinity Ava for your beautiful contributions. And to Laura Amazzone—in many ways, your book supercharged this book. To Sharon Gannon, for being my first experience of a yogini, and for showing me what kindness and humility look like. I will never forget you telling me that it was an "honor for you to be a part of my work."

To Kimberly Leo and Namaste Yoga in Oakland, for giving me a teaching platform. To Erik Singer and Prana del Mar retreat—thank you for your generosity with me, and your support. You are a true yogini haven. To Stuart Sovatsky, PhD for holding the lineage of the twilight language.

To Myrita Craig for believing in this book from day one with such resolve that I began to believe as well. And for flying cross-country to cook me soups and haul my crappy furniture to the curb. To Sally Grace Branch and the whole Branch family for their beautiful retreat river house, where some of this book was written, as well as their continual presence and support. To Meredith Hogan and the Shakti Factory for housing me in the Squirrel's Red Tent on countless occasions. Mer, your generosity and commitment to light is fueling much of the city of Cincinnati. And for your continual yogini support—Jill Loftis, Jessica Durivage Kerridge, Kim Garrison, Hollace Stephenson, Marcee Gutman Ballantyne, Nova Andrea Loverro, Kate Maxey, Kimber Simpkins, Hannah Webb Franco, Miranda Barrett, Sue Neufeld, Kathy O'Rourke, Daphne Larkin, Brenna Geehan, Katy Knowles, YogaTree San Francisco, Uttara Yoga in Roanoke, Virginia, and the entire Para Yoga community.

To the San Francisco Bay Area spiritual community for just existing, wearing your crazy costumes, and doing all the wild spirit-science-mind-body-eco-technological work that just keeps pushing the envelope and opening us all into new possibilities.

To all my other teachers, mentors, and inspirations—pranams—Dr. Vasant Lad, Dr. Claudia Welch, Devi Mueller, Andrey Lappa, Dr. Marc Halpern, Sandhiya Ramaswamy, A.G. and Indra Mohan, Javier Castro Alonso, Prashanti de Jager, Dr. David Frawley, Dr. Robert Svoboda, and Pandit Rajmani Tigunait.

To all my students—for your love, support, and your practice. I look forward to watching your evolution into Her.

And, finally, to people who read acknowledgement sections in books—you know who you are.

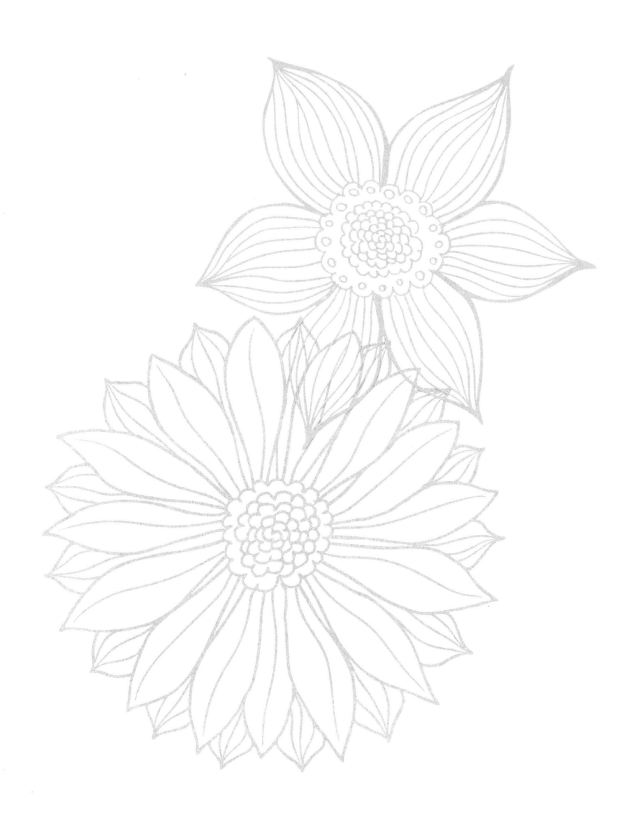

Appendix A

Open-Secret Recipes

This entire book has been a how-to overview on Ayurvedic living. Now it's time to bring Healthy, Happy, Sexy into the kitchen! In this section, I'm giving you some of my favorite happy-belly, Ayurveda-inspired recipes. There are millions of recipes I could have thrown in here, but these are a tasting, an overview of some basic, seasonal meals that will help you get lots of good whole-foods, plant-based, organic nutrition going in your life. Many of these recipes were experienced in the kitchens of my best buds and Ayurveda compatriots. These foods have been shared on many an occasion in my life. These soups were eaten in winter snowstorms with family members, at ocean-side yoga retreats on hot sunny days, and, most important, were brought to me by friends in moments of grief and sadness. Food heals. And this section will teach you how to become a healer.

Your new Ayurvedic lifestyle is going to require lots of cooked veggies, good fats, immune-boosting spices, whole grains, and seasonal fruits. When navigating your local grocery store, remember, the healthy stuff is usually on the edges of the grocery store (fruits, vegetables, bulk grains, dairy, eggs, and so on). Most of these recipes require almost nothing from the center of your supermarket (usually the realm of packages, cans, and jars).

The recipes are organized by season and doshic effect, making it super-easy for you to whip up an Ayurveda-inspired meal plan for any time of the year. I hope they stain your heart and hands beet-red. Okay, let's start simmering!

Spring Menu

Kapha-Reducing

Breakfast

Cooked Amaranth

Lunch

Quinoa with Fresh Basil, Avocado, and
  Lime
Dandelion Greens with Lemon and Dill
Homemade Hummus

Dinner

Simple Spring Pea Soup
Spicy Roasted Cauliflower

Sweets and Beverages

Ginger-Lime Coconut Water
Green Lemonade

Breakfast

Cooked Amaranth

½ cup amaranth
2 cups water
½ teaspoon cinnamon powder
1 teaspoon raw honey
Sprinkling of dried cranberries

Add the amaranth to boiling water. Reduce heat to low and simmer for
20–25 minutes, or until the water is absorbed. Make sure to stir a few
times while it cooks, as amaranth sticks and burns easily. Once cooked,
top with cinnamon, raw honey, and dried cranberries, and serve.

Lunch

Quinoa with Fresh Basil, Avocado, and Lime

Highly nourishing, avocados are good for building ojas. This is a great
summer dish: the grain is light, and the lime and basil reduce the heaviness of the avocado. This recipe can also reduce kapha even more if you
leave out the avocado.

3 cups water
½ cup white, red, or black quinoa
⅛ teaspoon rock salt
¼ teaspoon cumin powder
¼ teaspoon black pepper
¼ cup chopped fresh basil
1 whole ripe avocado
2 tablespoons extra-virgin olive oil
1 small lime, juiced

Bring the water to a boil and the add quinoa and salt. Cook over medium
heat for about 30 minutes, or until the quinoa is puffy. Cut the avocado
in half, remove the pit, and slice the inner flesh into cubes before peeling.

Drain quinoa and fluff with a fork, adding cumin, black pepper, chopped basil, and salt to taste. Gently mix in the avocado, olive oil, and lime juice.

Dandelion Greens with Lemon and Dill

These seasonal greens might be a little harder to find, but they are usually available at farmers' markets in the spring. Given that spring is the time for cleansing, it makes sense that Nature offers up these kapha-pacifying bile clearers. Dandelion greens are really good for getting rid of bad types of cholesterol in the blood and for reducing excess water weight. In this recipe, lemon and spices help your belly digest these cooling bitter leaves. That said, if you have a strong vata imbalance, avoid eating them.

2 tablespoons extra-virgin olive oil
½ medium sweet onion, diced
⅛ teaspoon rock salt
1 clove garlic, chopped
½ pound dried dandelion greens
½ fresh lemon, juiced
Black pepper to taste
¼ teaspoon dried dill, or a few sprigs of fresh dill, finely chopped

Heat the olive oil and add the onions and half the salt. Sauté the onions until they are translucent. Add the garlic. Meanwhile, blanch the greens in a medium-sized pot by placing them into boiling water for 1–2 minutes. Drain the excess water and finely chop the greens. Toss together with the onions, adding the fresh lemon juice and pepper. Garnish with dill.

Homemade Hummus

2 cups cooked chickpeas
½ lemon, juiced
2–3 tablespoons tahini
2 cloves garlic, crushed

½ teaspoon salt

3 tablespoons olive oil

Combine the ingredients in a blender or food processor. Blend for a few minutes on low, until thoroughly mixed and smooth. If the hummus is too thick, add a little water or olive oil. Garnish with fresh parsley or a dash of cayenne pepper.

Dinner

Simple Spring Pea Soup

2 teaspoons sunflower or olive oil

4 spring onions, finely minced

1 leek, chopped

1 cup vegetable or chicken stock

1½ cups fresh peas, shelled

1 teaspoon lemon juice

Salt and pepper to taste

In a small saucepan, sauté the spring onions and leek over medium-low heat for about 2 minutes, until translucent. Add the stock and bring to a boil. Add the peas and cook until bright green and slightly tender. (This depends on their size, but should only take a few moments.)

Using a blender, purée the soup until very smooth. Add the lemon juice and season with salt and pepper to taste. Drizzle a little extra-virgin olive oil on top or add a dab of yogurt for garnish. Serve warm or chilled.

Spicy Roasted Cauliflower

2 tablespoons olive oil or ghee

1 teaspoon roasted cumin powder

1 teaspoon chipotle powder, chili flakes, chili powder, or cayenne

Big pinch of salt

Black pepper to taste

1 medium cauliflower head, cut into small florets

Preheat the oven to 425°F. In a large mixing bowl, combine the oil, cumin powder, chipotle powder, salt, and pepper. Add the cauliflower to the bowl of seasoned oil and toss to thoroughly coat. Spread the mixture on a large baking sheet and roast for 25–40 minutes. Stir occasionally to ensure even browning.

Beverages

Ginger-Lime Coconut Water

10–12 ounces fresh coconut water (organic and bottled is also fine)
½ lime, juiced
1-inch chunk of fresh, unpeeled ginger
Pinch of cardamom powder (optional)

Mix the coconut water, lime juice, and ginger in a blender. You can also just grate the ginger and stir all ingredients together by hand. Add the cardamom on top for extra spice!

Green Lemonade

2-inch chunk of fresh peeled ginger
1 whole lemon, juiced
3 cups spinach
2 apples (Granny Smith for tart flavor or a red variety for sweet flavor)
Combine all ingredients in a juicer. Stir and drink.

Summer Menu

Pitta-Reducing

Breakfast
Coconut Chia Pudding
Date Smoothie

Lunch
Pistachio Rose Rice with Saffron
Simple Avocado and Arugula Salad
Green Goddess Soup

Dinner
Summer Tabouleh
Saffron Asparagus

Sweets and Beverages
Lavender-Infused Almond Smoothie
Greens Smoothie
Cucumber Mint Medicine Water

Breakfast

Coconut Chia Pudding

2 cups unsweetened coconut milk

⅓ cup chia seeds

¼ cup coconut flakes

3 tablespoons pistachios

Maple syrup or agave nectar to taste

¼ teaspoon cardamom powder

Handful organic rose petals, fresh or dried (optional garnish)

In a medium-sized bowl or large jar, stir together the coconut milk, chia seeds, coconut flakes, pistachios, maple syrup or agave nectar, and cardamom. Chill in the refrigerator for a few hours or until the chia seeds are expanded and soft. Before serving, stir once and spoon into serving dishes. Garnish with rose petals (if you have them) and enjoy.

Date Smoothie

1 teaspoon coconut oil

4–5 whole pitted dates

1 cup organic milk or almond milk

¼ teaspoon cardamom powder

¼ teaspoon cinnamon powder

2 tablespoons coconut flakes

Melt the coconut oil in a saucepan over low heat. Add the spices and coconut flakes, and warm them until they become aromatic. Be careful that they do not burn. Then, add milk. Whisk the spices into the milk and bring to a boil, cooking until foamy. Turn off heat. Pour the mixture into a blender and blend until smooth and liquid.

Lunch

Pistachio Rose Rice with Saffron

Good for reducing both pitta and vata, roses are said to reduce inflammation, heal a broken heart, and calm pitta on both the emotional and physical levels. Saffron is a known aphrodisiac, and good for building ojas and sattva in the mind.

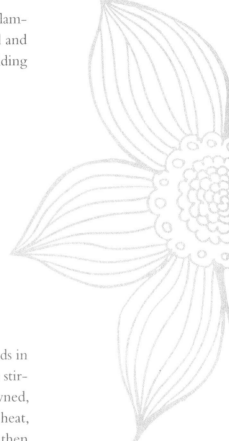

3 cups plus 4 tablespoons water
¼ teaspoon saffron
1 cup brown or basmati rice
2 tablespoons ghee
½ cup pistachios
¼ cup golden raisins
¼ teaspoon cooking-grade rose water
¼ teaspoon cooking-grade rose petals (dried or fresh)
¼ teaspoon cardamom powder
¼ teaspoon rock salt

Bring 3 cups of water to a boil and set aside. Place the saffron strands in 4 tablespoons of room-temperature water. In a dry sauté pan, while stirring frequently, toast the rice over medium heat until slightly browned, then add ghee. Remove from heat. In a separate pan over medium heat, dry-toast the chopped pistachios for 5 minutes or until browned, then add the raisins. If the boiled water has cooled too much, bring it back to a boil. Combine rice, pistachios, rose water, saffron water, cardamom, and rock salt with the boiled water. Cover and cook on low heat for about 30 minutes, or until the rice is cooked. Garnish with rose petals.

Simple Avocado and Arugula Salad

1 pound of arugula
6–8 dried apricots
¼ cup slivered almonds, skins removed
¼ cup Parmesan cheese

2 tablespoons extra-virgin olive oil

2 tablespoons lime juice or a sprinkle of sweet balsamic vinegar

Salt and pepper to taste

1 ripe avocado, cubed

Wash the arugula and chop or tear the leaves into bite-sized pieces. Place in a medium-sized mixing bowl. Slice the apricots thinly. Combine apricots, almonds, and cheese with the arugula. Whisk the oil and lime juice or vinegar together and pour the dressing onto the salad, along with salt and pepper to taste. Just before serving, top the salad with the avocado.

Green Goddess Soup

1 pound asparagus

1 tablespoon olive oil

Salt and freshly ground pepper to taste

2 teaspoons ghee

2 shallots, minced

1¼ cups chicken stock

3 cups organic arugula or other baby leafy greens

4 teaspoons whole-milk yogurt

Balsamic vinegar or truffle oil drizzled

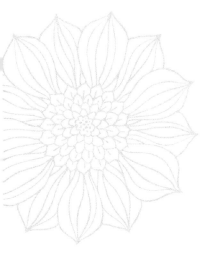

Preheat oven to 450°F. Snap off ends of the asparagus spears. Place the asparagus on a baking sheet and toss with olive oil, salt, and pepper. Roast in the oven for about 10 minutes or until the spears turn bright green but are still slightly crunchy. Shake the pan and continue roasting for a few more minutes, or until the asparagus begins to blacken. Cool and cut into 2-inch pieces.

In a medium pan, melt the ghee over medium heat. Add shallots and sauté until translucent. Add the asparagus and cook for 2–3 minutes. Stir in the stock, raise the heat to high, and boil for a few minutes. Add the greens and cook for 2–3 minutes. Remove from heat. Let the soup cool slightly, and pour into blender. Working in batches if necessary, purée until smooth. A handheld immersion blender also works well. Once pureed, divide into bowls and top each serving with a dollop of yogurt and a sprinkle of balsamic vinegar or truffle oil.

Dinner

Summer Tabouleh

1 cup water
½ cup organic cracked bulgur wheat
Salt and pepper to taste
4 plum tomatoes, finely diced
1 small sweet onion, chopped
1 medium cucumber, diced
2 large bunches of flat leaf parsley, finely chopped
10 fresh sprigs of mint, finely chopped
1 large lime (or 2 small limes), juiced
¼ cup extra-virgin olive oil
Optional: pitted kalamata olives, feta cheese, pan-roasted sunflower seeds, pumpkin seeds

In a medium pan, bring 1 cup water to a boil, then immediately remove from heat. Stir in bulgur wheat and cover. Let stand for 20–25 minutes to cook the grain. Meanwhile, salt the chopped tomatoes, and pepper the chopped onions. Mix the tomatoes and onions with the cucumber, parsley, mint, lime juice, and olive oil in a large serving bowl. Add the cooked grain to the mixture and blend well. Add more salt and pepper, if desired.

Saffron Asparagus

This is a great dish for early summer. Both asparagus and saffron purify the blood and are cooling and easy to digest.

5 strands of saffron
¼ teaspoon celery seeds (optional)
¼ teaspoon cumin seeds

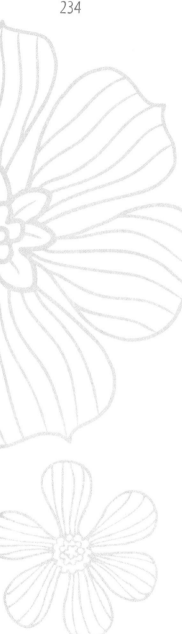

¼ teaspoon coriander seeds

2 tablespoons ghee

2 cups fresh asparagus, diced

⅛ teaspoon rock salt

¼ teaspoon fresh ground black pepper

¼ lemon, juiced

Grind the saffron with a mortar and pestle. Add a few drops of water and continue grinding until the saffron is dissolved, making a golden-hued water. Let stand for 5 minutes. Over medium heat, sauté the celery seeds, cumin, and coriander in ghee. Lower the heat just as the seeds begin to pop and release their aroma. Do not let them brown. Add the asparagus, salt, and pepper to the seed mixture. Then, add the saffron water and sauté until cooked. The mixture should be soft with a slight crunch. Once cooked, toss with the lemon juice and serve.

Beverages

Lavender-Infused Almond Smoothie

This is my attempt to bring together all of my favorite juicy-lady ingredients. Both sesame and almonds are highly revered for their ojas-building properties. Lavender cools and calms the nervous system. This is a great morning smoothie, although it can also be enjoyed as an afternoon snack.

3 tablespoons white or black sesame seeds

1/16 teaspoon dried lavender buds (food grade)

1 teaspoon maple syrup

1 cup almond milk

1–2 drops food grade rose essential oil (optional)

Roast the sesame seeds in a pan. In a coffee grinder, grind the seeds and lavender buds.

Combine the maple syrup and almond milk in a blender. Add the rose essential oil and the ground sesame and lavender. Blend and serve.

Greens Smoothie

1 large cucumber (peeled if not organic)

2 stalks celery

1 cup parsley

1 pear or apple

1-inch chunk fresh peeled ginger root

Place all ingredients in a blender. Blend on high until smooth. Drink first thing in the morning for a beautiful, anti-inflammatory tonic.

Cucumber Mint Medicine Water

1 small cucumber, thinly sliced

10–20 whole mint leaves

12 cups water

Rinse cucumber and mint. Combine in a large pitcher. Cover with water and refrigerate for at least 4 hours, or overnight. Serve at room temperature. Makes 1 gallon.

Fall/Early Winter Menu

Vata-Reducing

Breakfast

Oatmeal

Stewed Prunes

Lunch

Brown Rice with Nettles, Lemon, and Pine
  Nuts

Orange Velvety Beet Mash

Mary's Slow-Cooked Carrots and Leeks

Dinner

Immune-Boosting Pecan Soup

Sesame-Lime Sweet Potato Spinach Mash

Sweets and Beverages

Raw Chocolate Pudding

Mary Thompson's Chai

Breakfast

Oatmeal

A good warming breakfast, oats are one of the best foods for building ojas.

¾ cup whole oats
½ red apple, cored and chopped
1–2 pitted dates
¾ water
¾ cup almond milk
Toasted almonds, walnuts, or pecans
1 tablespoon Ghee or olive oil
Cinnamon, to taste

In a saucepan over medium heat, cook oats, apple, and dates in water and almond milk until soft. While oats are simmering, toast the nuts by roasting them over medium heat in a cast-iron pan, or any good skillet. Add a little ghee or olive oil to get them beautifully browned. When the oats are soft, add the cinnamon. The dates are so sweet, you usually won't need any sweetener!

Stewed Prunes

You can also use apples, apricots, pears, and cherries (as many fruits as you like!) in this beautifully warming winter fruit stew.

1 cup pitted prunes
1 cup dried cherries
½ teaspoon cinnamon powder
¼ teaspoon cardamom powder
Pinch of nutmeg powder
2–4 cups water

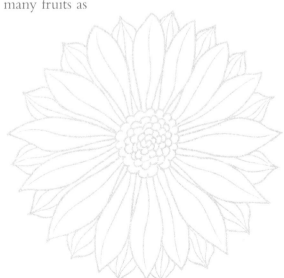

Combine all ingredients in a medium saucepan and bring to a boil. Reduce the heat and simmer for about 15 minutes. Enjoy the fruit by itself or as a topping for oatmeal. Reserve the extra liquid for desserts, or even drink as a tea.

Lunch

Brown Rice with Nettles, Lemon, and Pine Nuts

This is one of my all-time favorite dishes. Nettles tonify the blood, lemon stimulates digestion, and pine nuts are the best for treating cravings for savory foods. I eat this heavy dish when I'm craving macaroni and cheese. If you make this receipe with basmati rice instead of brown, it also reduces pitta. This goes well with a poached egg or a slice of smoked salmon.

> ¼ teaspoon mustard seeds
>
> ¼ teaspoon coriander seeds
>
> 2 tablespoons olive oil
>
> 1 small sweet yellow onion, chopped
>
> 1 cup brown rice
>
> 3 cups water
>
> ¼ cup dried nettles (available in most health food stores and online)
>
> 2 tablespoons pine nuts
>
> ⅛ teaspoon rock salt
>
> ¼ teaspoon fresh ground black pepper
>
> ½–1 lemon
>
> Feta cheese or pesto (optional garnish)

Sauté the seed spices in the oil until aromatic. Add onions and sauté until translucent. Next, add the brown rice and continue to cook for another minute, stirring. Add water, nettles, and bring to a medium boil. In a separate pan, sauté the pine nuts and remaining ingredients. When soft, remove the rice from heat. Drain any excess water.

Garnish with black pepper, feta cheese, or pesto and serve.

Orange Velvety Beet Mash

A wonderful winter blood builder.

½ medium onion, finely chopped

¼ teaspoon rock salt

¼ teaspoon fennel seeds

1 teaspoon ghee or olive oil

3 medium or large organic beets, peeled and chopped

1 large sweet potato, chopped

2 tablespoons coconut oil

1 tablespoon maple syrup

1 small orange, juiced

Coconut, grated (optional garnish)

In a deep, heavy-bottomed saucepan, sauté the onions, salt, and fennel seeds in ghee or olive oil. Add the beets and sweet potato and sauté at medium heat for about 1 minute. Cover with water until beets and sweet potato are submerged and bring to a boil, cooking until softened. Drain and mash, stirring in the coconut oil, maple syrup, and orange juice. Garnish with grated coconut for added beauty.

Mary's Slow-Cooked Carrots and Leeks

1 medium sweet yellow onion or 2–3 shallots, finely chopped

1 clove garlic, minced

3 tablespoons ghee or olive oil

Salt and pepper to taste

3 large carrots, thinly sliced (about quarter-sized)

1 large leek, washed and thinly sliced

1 fresh lemon, juiced

Handful of parsley, finely chopped

A few sprigs of dill, finely chopped

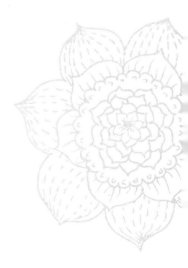

Sauté the onions and garlic in the olive oil and salt on medium until translucent. Add the carrots and leeks and cook for a few minutes, stirring occasionally. Reduce heat to low, cover, and cook for 20–30 minutes. Once the carrots are soft and slightly caramelized, turn off the heat. Add the lemon juice, fresh parsley, and dill. Mix and serve.

Dinner

Immune-Boosting Pecan Soup

This warming soup is protein-rich and helps boost our defenses during the winter months.

> 1 large yellow onion, chopped
> 2 tablespoons olive or sesame oil
> Pinch of salt
> 2 cloves garlic, minced
> 1 tablespoon cayenne or chili powder
> 4 sprigs fresh thyme
> 1 bay leaf
> 3 cups raw pecans
> 3 cups vegetable broth
> 1 cup organic plain soy cream
> ¼ cup maple syrup
> ¼ cup chopped fresh scallions or cilantro

In a deep pot, sauté the onions in olive oil and salt. Once the onions are translucent, add the garlic and continue stirring for 1 minute, until golden. Turn the heat to low and add the spices and pecans. Stir to combine fully. Add the broth and bring to a boil. Turn the heat down and simmer for 30 minutes. Turn off the heat and let the soup cool. Once lukewarm, pour the mixture into a blender and puree. Return the soup back to the pot and reheat, adding the soy cream and maple syrup slowly. Continue stirring until mixture is creamy. Serve hot with cilantro or scallions for garnish.

Sesame-Lime Sweet Potato Spinach Mash

A mouthful to say, but it's an even bigger fullness to the taste.

  4 sweet potatoes, chopped
  ¼ cup coconut shavings
  6 tablespoons sesame seeds
  ¼ teaspoon rock salt
  1 pound of fresh spinach, well-washed and chopped
  1 tablespoon ghee or olive oil
  1 lime, juiced
  1 teaspoon toasted sesame oil

Boil the sweet potatoes until soft. (I wash them well and leave the skins on for added nutrients, but you can also peel them for better mouth-feel.) In a cast-iron pan or skillet, roast the coconut shavings, sesame seeds, and salt until golden brown. Remove from pan and set aside. Sauté the spinach in the ghee or olive oil until soft and bright green. Once potatoes are soft, strain and mash. Stir the cooked spinach into the mash. Drizzle with lime juice and toasted sesame oil. Sprinkle with the sesame-coconut mix.

Dessert

Raw Chocolate Pudding

This exotic raw food pudding requires good digestive health and is highly addictive, so enjoy in moderation. I was inspired by Cafe Gratitude's Raw Cacao Smoothie, but added my own twist. Enjoy!

  1 cup water
  2 dates, pitted
  ½ avocado
  2 fresh figs (or 2 dates if figs are not in season)

1 tablespoon cacao butter

2 tablespoons raw cacao powder

⅛ teaspoon vanilla extract

¼ cup brazil nuts

Combine all ingredients into a blender or food processor and blend until smooth.

Beverages

Mary Thompson's Chai

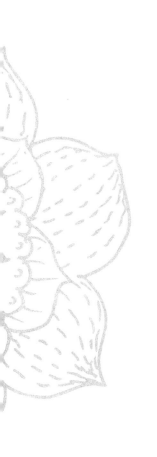

10 cups water

3 teaspoons of ginger, powdered or freshly grated

3 teaspoons cardamom powder

4 teaspoons cinnamon, powdered or freshly grated

2 teaspoons fennel seeds

1 teaspoon coriander seeds

½ teaspoon nutmeg, powdered or freshly grated

½ teaspoon whole cloves

Pinch of black pepper

3–5 teaspoons black tea (depending on how strong you like it)

Honey, Sucanat, or raw cane sugar to taste

½ gallon whole milk, oat milk, or soy milk

Slowly boil (decoct) all the herbs and spices in a medium to large pot in 10 cups of water. Do NOT add the black tea yet. Reduce this mixture down to about 8 cups. Turn off the heat and add black tea. Stir, cover the pot and let sit for no more than 10 minutes (any more than that and the tea will become bitter). Strain mixture and add milk. Heat again until the new mixture becomes hot but not boiling. Sweeten with honey, Sucanat, or raw cane sugar to taste. Add a tiny sprinkling of nutmeg to each cup of hot chai. For a special peppermint chai, add equal parts of peppermint leaf when adding the black tea.

Kitchari—The Answer to All Your Belly's Woes

Kitchari is good for all doshic types and can be tailored to the seasons when spiced appropriately. Basmati rice and mung dal are sweet, cooling, and easy on the digestion. Kitchari is a complete food, said to nourish the tissues, boost strength, and increase our vitality. It is also the preferred food we use when doing any type of deep cleansing. Here are three seasonal kitchari recipes.

Summer (Pitta-Reducing) Kitchari

Use this anytime you have a pitta imbalance, such as acid indigestion or inflammation. It is also a great dish to serve weekly for any dosha during the hottest months of the year.

1 cup yellow mung dal (whole mung beans are fine if you can't get split)
1 cup basmati rice
1½-inch piece of fresh ginger, peeled and minced
¼ cup shredded unsweetened coconut
½ cup fresh cilantro
3 tablespoons ghee or coconut oil
½ teaspoon fennel seeds
½ teaspoon coriander seeds
½ teaspoon cumin seeds
1 teaspoon turmeric
½ teaspoon salt
6 cups water
Garnish with 2 tablespoons shredded coconut and cilantro

Wash and rinse the dal and rice until water is clear. Soaking the dal for a few hours before cooking will make it more digestible. Put the ginger, coconut, cilantro, and ½ cup water into a blender and blend until liquified. In a large saucepan over medium heat, heat the ghee, then add the fennel, cumin, and coriander seeds. Stir until fragrant, about 1 minute. Add turmeric, salt, and the blended liquid. Stir for a few minutes, then add the mung and rice, and mix well. Pour in the water, cover, and bring to a medium boil. Let boil for 5 minutes, then turn down the heat to very low. Cook, lightly covered, until the dal and rice are soft, about 25–30 minutes.

Meanwhile, toast the coconut in an iron pan or skillet until brown. When done, the beans and rice will have a porridge texture. Garnish with the coconut and a little fresh cilantro. Note: If you prefer, use half the water, and cook the mung beans with the spices and the rice separately, in a rice cooker.

Fall Kitchari (Vata-Reducing)

Follow the same recipe as above, but replace the coconut, fennel, and coriander with cinnamon, black pepper, mustard seeds, ajwan seeds, and hing. You can use any combination of these spices, or all of them. Use this anytime you have a vata imbalance, such as bloating, gas, or dryness. It is also a great weekly dish during the coldest months of the year.

Spring Kitchari (Kapha-Reducing)

Follow the same recipe as above, but replace the coconut, fennel, and coriander with cinnamon, black pepper, cloves, bay leaves, and ginger powder. You can use all of these ingredients or any combination of them. Use this anytime you have a kapha imbalance, such as mucous conditions or a feeling that you ate too much fatty or fried food the day before.

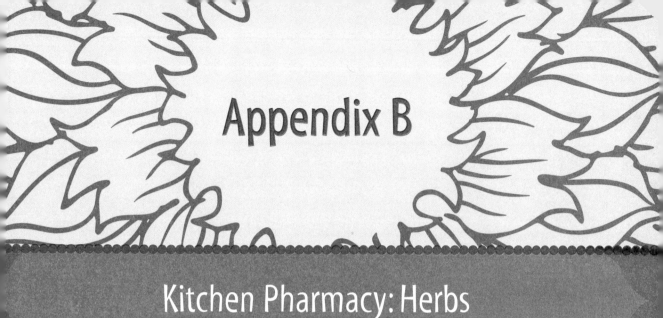

Appendix B

Kitchen Pharmacy: Herbs

I am a fan of playing with plants. I learn about them one by one. I buy them, smell them, chop them, store them in pretty jars, and pretend I am a kitchen witch who has no fear of the Inquisition. I even meditate with the herbs. I hold them in my hands and say, "Hey, pretty darling. Thank you. Whisper to me what you can do, and I will do my best to protect you."

Many plants can be used to support core vitality. This section includes some basic herbal remedies for common imbalances. Many of these herbs and food remedies are found in your kitchen. The more obscure herbs can be easily purchased from the online retailers listed in the resources section. All herbs are powerful, and should not be used willy-nilly. These herbs are meant to be used as a support for your body's natural immunity, not necessarily to cure an acute disease or problem.

Kitchen-Pharmacy Remedies

Sleep Tonics

Sweet Dreams Milk: This is a milky beverage that counteracts insomnia and nervousness before bed. You can also enhance the effects of this milky medicine by rubbing some warm sesame oil and a few drops of jatamamsi essential oil on the soles of your feet before covering in socks.

1 teaspoon ghee
½ teaspoon valerian powder
½ teaspoon ashwaghanda powder
Dash of nutmeg powder
A few strands of saffron
1 cup whole milk, almond milk, soy
  milk, or hazelnut milk

Put the ghee in a saucepan and heat on low with all the spices, except for the saffron. Once the mixture becomes aromatic, add the milk and saffron and whisk until hot.

Cold and Flu Support

- **Steamy Sinus Relief:** To relieve sinus congestion, boil a large pot of water. Once boiling, remove the pot from the stovetop, add 5 drops of eucalyptus and cover with a towel. Put your head under the towel to breathe in the steam. You can also add a couple teaspoons of dried ginger powder for extra heat and decongestion support.
- **Sore Throat Gargle:** Mix ½ teaspoon of turmeric with ½ teaspoon sea salt in warm water. Gargle. You can also dab the back of your throat with 1–2 small drops of neem oil.
- **Sore Throat Nectar:** Mix 2 tablespoons of turmeric with some local honey (if available) and the juice of half a lemon. Mix until it makes a nice paste. You can take 1 teaspoon a few times a day. Add some black pepper, ginger powder, or cinnamon if you feel cold in your body. If you are getting over bronchitis, or want to strengthen your lungs, mix the turmeric with equal parts ghee and honey. Add ½ teaspoon black pepper and ¼ teaspoon ginger and make a paste. Eat a teaspoon of this 5–6 times a day.
- **Classic Lemon Ginger Honey:** This is one of the best remedies for the cruddy feeling of a cold coming on. On many a cold Virginia night, I have taken this and woke up feeling fine. Slice a thumb-sized amount of fresh ginger and simmer 1 to 2 cups water on medium-low for 15–30 minutes. Once the ginger-water has cooled, add some lemon and honey. Keep the water lukewarm if using honey, as "cooked" honey is harder for the body to digest. High temperatures kill its medicinal properties.

Sexual Vitality Support

Whipped into a Frenzy

This is a super easy edible butter for igniting sexual juiciness. (Note: There are a number of reasons why the vagina doesn't emit secretions, but typically constipation, irregular menstruation, and stress accompany this problem. Speak to a qualified Ayurvedic practitioner to assess any deeper imbalances that may be emotional or mental in nature. A woman's juiciness may also dry up if she is with a man she does not love or trust; if she feels resentful toward him; if she has feelings for someone else; or if she is feeling guilty.) To activate your sensual feminine energy, do some deep belly breathing and the Breathe into Your Roots meditation from page 209 to increase energy in this area. Then, make this:

2 tablespoons powdered licorice
2 tablespoons ghee
2 tablespoons uncooked organic honey (local if possible)
1 teaspoon shatavari powder
½ teaspoon cardamom powder
½ teaspoon ashwaghanda powder

Blend all ingredients until a paste forms. Take ½ teaspoon 2–3 times daily, or 1 teaspoon a few hours before lovemaking.

Tea for Boosting Sensual Flow

The juiciness of the body can dry up when the nervous system lacks nourishment. This time-tested combination is a nervine tonic, relaxing constriction and promoting blood flow. It also kindles the sensitivity of our nerve endings, allowing for us to be more receptive and sensitive to the touch of our beloved. Energetically, wild oat and damiana support a woman's sexual openness, promoting better lovemaking, as well as personal healing around sexual trauma. All of these ingredients are mild nervine tonifiers and help to promote relaxation and ease.

4 parts wild oat
2 parts damiana
2 parts lemon balm
1 part licorice root shavings or powder
1 part gingerroot powder
1 part shatavari powder

Combine all ingredients and store in an airtight glass container. When needed, make a tea out of the mixture using 1–3 tablespoons, steeped for 10–15 minutes in boiling water.

Simple Remedies to Restore Core Vitality and Womb Happiness

- **The PMS bath:** For a stress-soothing soak before your period starts, take a PMS bath. Start by giving yourself a nice oil massage with the appropriate oil for your constitutional type (page 141). Fill the bath and put in 3 drops clary sage, 3 drops lavender, and 2 drops rose absolute or attar. Lavender, chamomile, and rose geranium are also excellent for relieving emotional stagnation and opening the heart. Massage your belly in a clockwise motion.
- **For headaches:** Eat a light dinner, such as a soup or brothy stew and do nasya before bed (page 129). For sharp, intense headaches that are accompanied by pressure and heat, make a sandalwood and aloe paste and apply to your forehead and neck. Leave for 20 minutes, then rinse.
- **For general uterine health:** A warm castor oil compress helps reduce stagnation in the flow of menstrual blood. You can do this 3–4 times a week for 30–60 days, except when you are menstruating. In severe cases, when a woman is experiencing very irregular periods, or a total cessation of menstruation, this can be done daily for 30–60 days. You will need a large plastic bag, several rags or towels that you do not mind getting a little oily, and a hot water bottle. Lie down. Pour approximately ⅛ cup castor oil

on your lower abdomen, from your belly button to pubic bone. Cover with towels and then with the plastic bag. Place hot water compress on the bag and let sit for at least 90 minutes. Relax and enjoy.[1]

- **For a hot vagina:** If your lady bits are feeling hot or itchy, try this ancient technique for cooling off your hot spot. Soak a 1" × 3" clean cotton cloth in pure, unprocessed, organic coconut oil and place into your vagina before you go to bed. You can also do it for a few hours during the day. It's best to do this 3–5 days prior to your period. Do not do this practice if you have any other vaginal issues, such as a yeast infection, sores, and so forth. You can also soak a nontoxic, organic cotton tampon in coconut oil. Add 4–6 drops of pure neem oil, 5 drops of rose essential oil, and 10 drops of lavender essential oil. Insert for 2–4 hours, or overnight.

- **For excessive flow:** Ayurveda author and expert Dr. Vasant Lad recommends taking 1–2 teaspoons of a combination of raspberry and hibiscus flowers as a tea.[2]

- **To balance flow all month long:** All doshas can benefit from the juicy goodness of the feminine goddess of all plants, aloe vera. Take 1 tablespoon of pure aloe vera gel orally (organic, no additives) the week before your period, 3 times a day.

- **For yeast infections:** This common bummer situation can usually be remedied easily if caught early. You do not need to run to the pharmacy! One note of caution: some people are extremely sensitive to tea tree oil. In general, we don't put certain essential oils on the body (e.g., clove, cinnamon, or any of the sage family), but tea tree is usually well tolerated by most people. To make sure, first rub a tiny amount of the solution on your vaginal walls. You will feel a light burning or stinging, but it should go away in a few minutes. If the burning doesn't stop in less than a few minutes, your skin may be too sensitive for this remedy. If you tolerate the oil, take one organic cotton all-natural tampon (the small kind, without the cardboard applicator). Mix about 1 teaspoon

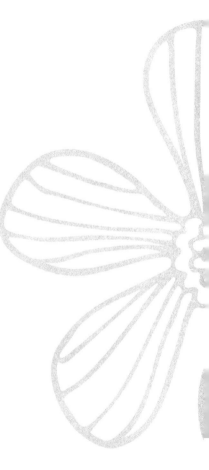

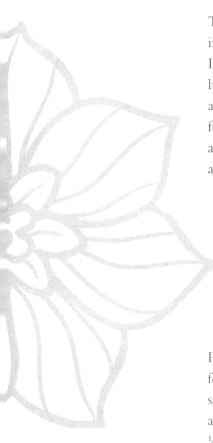

of sesame or coconut oil with equal amounts of tea tree oil. Roll the tampon in this solution and insert. It's best to use it at night and go to sleep with the tampon inside. Do not use the remedy if you are already menstruating.

Strong Body/Happy Mind Tonics

Golden Mama Milk

This is my remedy for the 10:00 PM "I really wanna hot fudge sundae in bed" cravings. In fact, I experienced a dramatic shift in my life when I stopped eating after sunset and replaced a heavy dinner with a super light liquid one. Sometimes, if I eat a good strong lunch and a light late afternoon snack, I replace dinner with this Yogini Milk. It makes me feel full-on self-love and nurturance. It contributes to better sleep and a clear mind upon waking. It is also an antioxidant-rich remedy for anxious sleeping.

    1 teaspoon ghee
    ½ teaspoon turmeric powder
    ¼ teaspoon cardamom powder
    Pinch of nutmeg powder
    A few strands of saffron
    1 cup whole milk, almond milk, soy milk, or hazelnut milk

Put the ghee in a saucepan over low heat with all the spices except for the saffron. Once the mixture becomes aromatic, add the milk and saffron and whisk until hot. You can also throw this into a blender for a frothier hot milk. To make this more of a rejuvenating tonic, add ½ teaspoon shatavari or ashwaganda powder.

Yogini Rose Elixir

This cooling rose elixir soothes the mind, opens the heart, and kindles the flame of immunity.

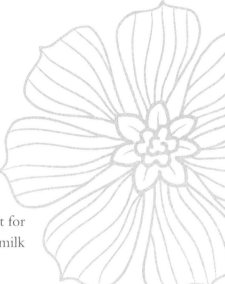

1 teaspoon ghee or coconut oil

½ teaspoon maple syrup

½ teaspoon brahmi powder

¼ teaspoon shatavari powder

¼ teaspoon cardamom powder

¼ teaspoon licorice powder

¼ teaspoon tulsi powder

2 drops pure rose attar essential oil

1 cup whole milk, almond milk, soy milk, or hazelnut milk

Put the ghee in a saucepan over low heat with all the spices except for the rose essential oil. Once the mixture becomes aromatic, add the milk and rose oil and whisk until hot.

Trinity's Golden Wonder Tea

Here is another yummy recipe from Trinity Ava. Take this if you have a cold or feel general weakness, or after you have done intense physical labor. This recipe was given to her by a wonderful yogi and mentor named Nanak Dave Singh. This tea is also highly beneficial for the lungs, as well as any pain, strain, or general trauma to the body. Drink 1–2 cups per day, as needed. This is a large amount of turmeric per day, so I don't recommend using this for longer than one week, or every other week as needed, if the issue is acute.

2 cups water

6 slices fresh gingerroot, sliced

4 tablespoons organic turmeric powder

1 tablespoon ghee

1 cup warm milk, coconut milk, or milk alternative or 1 cup ginger or tulsi (holy basil) tea (optional)

Honey to taste

Pinch of cardamom powder (to garnish)

Additional ingdredients for a cooling effect: gotu kola and goji berries (as many as you want)

Simmer water, ginger slices, and turmeric powder with 1 tablespoon of ghee for 30–45 minutes until it yields a golden-red paste. Add extra water, if needed. Add 1–2 tablespoons of the turmeric paste to warm organic milk, or ginger or tulsi tea. Add almond milk, hemp milk, or oat milk to taste. During the simmering phase, you could also add any of the following spices: 1 tablespoon ashwagandha powder, 6 fresh ginger slices, or ½ teaspoon ground black pepper. Strain well before drinking.

Add 2 tablespoons of ghee, honey to taste, milk or milk alternative, and a pinch of cardamom powder to your turmeric and tea or milk base. Drink with a spoon nearby to avoid the big chunk of turmeric paste at the bottom! Store any additional turmeric powder paste in the fridge until your next round of tea. If this formula of herbs is too heating for you, add cooling herbs, such as gotu kola or goji berries, to make the formula more constitutionally appropriate with herbs.

Bone Support

Strong Bones Broth

Bone broth helps us replenish trace minerals in the body, strengthening the bones and reducing vata. Excellent for vata women, women who are menstruating, or women in the menopausal or postmenopausal years. Ask your local butcher for organic chicken or beef bones, which you can store in the freezer.

Place several large bones in a large soup pot and cover with water. Add a splash of apple cider vinegar to extract more of the minerals from the broth. Bring to a boil and skim off any extra gristle that rises to the top. You can add a chopped carrot, onion, or celery if you want extra flavor. Lower the flame and simmer for 4–24 hours. The longer you simmer the broth, the more mineral-rich it will be! This bone-enriching medicine will last for a week in the fridge. You can also freeze it and use it for soups, stews, and rice dishes in the future.

Chyawanprash

I don't recommend trying to make this epic health-boosting lickable in your own home, as it contains no less than 46 herbs. Some mixtures contain over 100 herbs. Legend holds that the great sage Chyawana fell in love with a nubile young woman. Sad that he was an old man, he created this formula, reversed his age, and enjoyed her delights as a young virile stud. Have a couple of teaspoons every day when your digestion is strong. (See resources.)

Digestive Support

- **A general cure-all for digestive issues:** Take a piece of whole, unpeeled gingerroot and grate, reserving 2 teaspoons. Stir the ginger into a cup of hot water and let steep for 2 minutes. You can strain it, but I like drinking it with the gingerroot included. Fresh ginger tea also does wonders for general indigestion and flatulence.
- **For constipation:** Whether it's due to an imbalanced lifestyle, our constitutional makeup, or a lot of air travel, we all experience some form of constipation. In general, the best way to treat it is to clean up your diet, exercise, lay off the soda and caffeine, drink some herbal teas and warm water, and get on a regular food routine. Notice if you are rushing out the door instead of taking time to eliminate in the morning. Would you ask your pet to do that? Please, don't do it to yourself. Try taking 1 teaspoon of triphala before bed and upon rising. For bad constipation (especially while traveling), a quick remedy is to take 1 teaspoon of flax oil or castor oil before bed with some warm water. This has a mildly laxative effect on the system and is not meant to be used more than a few days. You can also soak a few prunes in water overnight. In the morning, drink the prune water or eat the prunes or both.
- **For indigestion:** Eat a few thin slices of ginger with a splash of lime and rock salt before meals.
- **For sluggish digestion:** Mix ⅛ teaspoon of salt, ⅛ teaspoon of ginger powder, and ⅛ teaspoon of black pepper in a spoon. Add a little lemon and take while you are preparing your meal. By the time lunch is ready, your digestive Fire will be ready. You can also take some trikatu, a common Ayurvedic digestive stimulant containing ginger, black pepper, and long pepper (a common Indian spice available in Indian shops and online).
- **For loose stools:** Amalaki is a great herb for reducing the amount of heat in the digestive tract and helping to firm stools. Take ½ teaspoon with warm water before bed nightly.

- **For gas and bloating due to excess air:** Mix equal parts fennel seeds, ajwan seeds, and cumin seeds. Roast lightly. Chew about 1 teaspoon for relief from gas. You can store the rest in a glass container and use when needed.
- **For hyperacidity:** Mix equal parts fennel seeds, coriander seeds, and cumin seeds. Roast lightly. Chew about 1 teaspoon as needed.

Goddess, Meet Ghee

There is a love affair happening in my heart, and it is covered in ghee. Ghee is butter, slowly boiled so that all the milk solids can be removed. It's great for boosting metabolic Fire. In fact, it is as important to Ayurveda as lubrication is to sex. You can think of ghee as love oil for the body. This oily love nectar, made from milk, is a medicine. It is also an excellent carrier (anupana) for herbs, helping your body absorb what the spices offer. Ghee lubricates your joints, tissues, muscles, hair, skin, nails, and vagina. Its healing capacities may lie in the process one has to go through to make it "from scratch," reducing milk to its golden essence. You can buy organic forms of ghee at your local health food store, but it is a sensual experience to connect to your ancient goddess-self by making it at home.

To enable you to truly understand the miracle of ghee and how it relates healing and our own Juicy Inner Feminine, I want to tell you a story. Imagine that once upon a time you were a hip mama living in 200 BC in India. There was no Ghee-Mart and there were no fitness centers. You got your Michelle Obama arms through the daily grind. As the sun rose and the cock crowed, you snuggled yourself up to milk Bessie, your cow. Afterward, you boiled her milk and allowed it to slowly cool. You added a yogurt culture to the milk and let it sour into a clabber. After a few days, you skimmed off the milk fat that had risen to the top, and began the laborious task of agitating the fat in a huge wooden churn.

After several hours of diligent churning (perhaps you traded off with your sister or cousin while chatting about the latest village goings-on), you would have not only a small vat of butter to show for your efforts, but also have completed your daily workout. This precious vat of butter—filled with all your hard work and girl-secrets—got simmered over the wood fire until all of the water had boiled out and the milk solids had risen to the top. You strained the solids off and kept what remained: clear, golden, pure love.

Making Ghee

Put 1 pound of unsalted, organic butter in a medium-sized pan and melt over medium heat. Once the butter is liquefied, turn down the

The Gifts that Ghee Has to Give

Here are some of the health-boosting properties of ghee that will turn you into an age-defying, glowing goddess. (Remember, ghee should be used in moderation. About ½–1 teaspoon per meal is good for most people.)

- Has powerful anti-inflammatory properties
- Boosts metabolism when taken with meals
- Highly stable cooking agent
- Balances all three doshas in moderation
- Acts as a carrier and synergy-food for other medicines and nutrients, supercharging their properties
- Is a nutritive tonic
- Is said to soothe a hoarse throat and smooth the voice
- Slows the aging process
- Fosters strength and resiliency
- Makes the skin smooth and luscious
- Is said to boost memory, intelligence, and decision-making abilities
- Softens and tones tissues, making it a great massage oil
- Soothes red, dry, or burning eyes
- Directly tones and supports the reproductive system in both women and men
- Is said to increase virility and libido in women and men
- Is used to brighten the complexion
- Is better than butter, because the milk solids (the stuff that clogs your arteries) have been removed in the cooking process

heat until the butter just boils. Cook uncovered at this temperature. Eventually, the butter will foam and bubble. White curds will burst to the surface of the foam and then float to the bottom of the pot. The ghee will start to smell amazing, like buttered popcorn. It will eventually turn a transparent, golden color. Keep the ghee on medium-low and monitor it often, as it can easily burn. You will know it's burning if it starts to turn a brown color and smell "nutty." Once golden and clear (the solids will have gone to the bottom), you can take a slatted spoon and strain off some of the foam. This will also allow you to see the "bottom" of the ghee. Make sure it's clear. Eventually, it will stop foaming and bubbling. This is a good sign that it's done. Remove from heat and let it cool before straining through a few layers of cheesecloth pressed over a fine strainer. Store in a dry glass jar with a lid. Throw out the leftover crunchy milk solids. Generally, I have found that each pound of butter takes about 20 minutes of cooking time. More butter will take longer.

Ghee can be kept on the kitchen counter in a glass jar at room temperature. It does not need refrigeration. Make sure to use a dry spoon when you use your ghee, as water in the jar can spoil and mold the ghee. Otherwise, it keeps for a really long time. Like, forever.

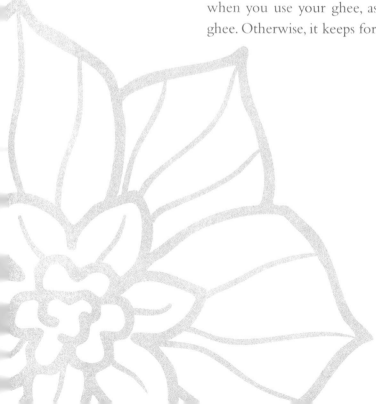

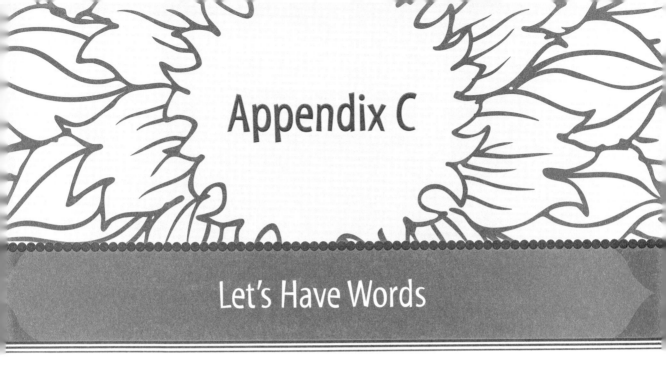

Appendix C

Let's Have Words

This section is based on statements and questions I hear from women all the time. It is also based on topics that seem to be sensitive for some of us; it's like an FAQ for your health and Ayurvedic questions.

A Word on Ghee, Butter, Other Oils, and Fats

Oh my God, are you seriously asking me to eat clarified butter (ghee)? Won't I get fat?

Appropriate amounts of ghee, butter, and other high-quality fats don't make you fat; they prevent you from getting fat. Fats are lipids, meaning they hold energy, stimulate digestion, and absorb toxins, allowing the gunk (ama) to more easily slide right on out of your body. Without fats, things get dry and stuck and sad and unsexy. And by the way, your brain is one beautifully plump chick! She is made up of 60

percent fat. Good-quality fats such as organic butter, hemp, flax, ghee, and olive oil, coconut oil, and fish oils have been shown to reduce the risk of breast cancer and improve heart health.[1] These oils can also help balance our hormones, lower the bad kind of cholesterol, and reduce our risk of heart attack. I know, it's the opposite of what we've been told. So eat these fats in moderation.

A Word on Chocolate

Chocolate is my 4:00 PM office lover.

I know. Me too. But just like any lover, you can get addicted. Are you eating it in moderation (like, a few little squares)? And is it organic and dark? Then, great. But has it become a daily habit to get you through the workday? Or has it become a replacement for spooning with your husband, with whom you feel a lack of intimacy lately? Maybe not so great. We crave chocolate as women because it's full of magnesium and zinc, which may get depleted with changes in our hormones. Studies show that chocolate has a chemical in it called phenethylamine. This chemical boosts the feelings of being in love: relaxation, mild euphoria, intoxication, and pleasure. Chocolate also releases mood-boosting, stress-reducing serotonin. Go rent the movie *Like Water for Chocolate* and eat a few squares. Just don't burn the house down with your passion for it.

A Word on Coffee

Want me to stop drinking espresso? You're gonna have to pull this latte out of my cold, dead hand!

Well, before we talk about coffee, let's first talk about rat orgasms. Yes, rat orgasms. There are actually experiments where the rat can lean up against an electrode bar that gives it a mild shock to the pleasure center in its brain. This causes the rat to instantly have an orgasm. The rat will lean up against the bar all day long. And after a day or so, the poor oversexed rodent just keels over dead in a pool of its own self-pleasure.

My mother's coffeemaker used to be my own personal orgasmatron. This decidedly delicious (and expensive) espresso maker grinds the beans before each little cup. It steams the milk. It tells me that my crusty morning-face looks lovely as it pours out the most addictive, nutty cuppa Joe with the press of one easy button. My addiction was all good until I learned about my ovaries and the special relationship between the coffee bean and the human female reproductive system (another kind of bean holder, if you will). According to Dr. Claudia Welch's book *Balance Your Hormones, Balance Your Life*, the coffee bean has a particular affinity with our lady parts. Coffee is typically sprayed with gnarly chemical pesticides that are by nature estrogenic (that is, they affect the female sex hormones). When we drink coffee, these chemicals concentrate in our breast tissue. Dr. Welch says that it also has an affinity with reproductive tissue in general.

The Standard American Diet (which you may recall as the SAD diet) is typically very heavy and mucus-forming. When things are harder to digest, our elimination gets stagnant and we reach for coffee as a mechanism to initially enhance peristalsis (i.e., the urge to go). Over time, though, coffee can progressively dry out the digestive system and weaken the colon. It is also highly acidic (pitta) in nature and dries out our tissues. And we want to stay juicy, remember?

If you really don't want to give up coffee, that's okay. I still indulge when I go to my mom's house or the occasional cafe. Just make sure you pay the extra cash and go organic, 100 percent of the time. You can also lower coffee's acidity by grinding some fresh cardamom and nutmeg into your beans. Also, try not to drink it black. Adding organic milk, nut milk, or cream, and a natural sweetener will lower its acidic effect.

A Word on Vegetarianism and Veganism

Do I have to go vegetarian to be Ayurvedic?

Nope, you can do whatever you want because *you are the boss*. Even great saints and spiritual beings have used meat as a medicine when they were ill. It is typical for an Ayurvedic doctor to prescribe bone-broth stews and a little stewy meat to patients who are depleted. Eating more veggies, grains, fruits, a little bit of the good fats, and the occasional organic dairy product will be better for your belly and create less negative karma for the world. That said, there is no doubt that a primarily vegetarian diet is more humane and creates less suffering (karma)—at least according to yoga, Ayurveda, science, and my mom.

A Word on White Rice

Is white rice bad for me?

That depends on which kind of white rice you eat. White jasmine rice, basmati rice, and brown rice are all staples in my Ayurveda-lovin' pantry. The white rice commonly found in supermarkets is energetically dead. It has been strip-mined of many of its vital nutrients. A good organic basmati, on the other hand, is light, tasty, easy for your body to digest, and nutritious. Basmati rice is a great food to turn to when your digestion feels sluggish, gassy, or acidic. Always rinse your rice before cooking, to pull off the first layer of gluten. For optimal digestibility, soak your rice (and all grains, for that matter) for at least 15–30 minutes before cooking. Then, sauté the rice in ghee until it turns translucent. You can also add some spices. Then go ahead and cook it in your rice cooker or steamer. I also like to add a few strips of kombu (a type of seaweed you can buy at health food stores) or dried astragalus strip to the boiling rice water for added immune boosting and nutrition. These little tricks will not only make your rice (and beans) yummier, it will help you digest it better.

A Word on Brown Rice

Is brown rice okay?

Totally. It's just heavier and a little harder to digest than whole-grain basmati rice, which is naturally white. If your digestive Fire is strong and you don't feel heavy, eat brown rice for its higher nutrition content. It is especially appropriate in the fall and winter.

A Word on Rice Cakes

Look how healthy I am, I eat rice cakes!

Okay, but—if I can get personal here—is your vagina dry? For women who love rice cakes, the answer is usually yes. Remember, you are what you eat. If you want to be a dry, rigid, stale cake, then eat them, but if you want to be juicy, go for a moist piece of fresh rye bread or, even better, a bowl of cinnamon-spiced butternut squash soup. Again, there are times when rice cakes may be appropriate, depending on the season, your imbalance, and your body type, but for most of the women I know, rice cakes lead to more flighty ungroundedness and an "I-feel-starved" post-digestive effect.

A Word on Mung Beans

I hate the sound of "mung beans"! Do I have to eat them?

Yes. The mung bean is majestic, and I can't wait for you two to become best friends. Also called "the sunshine bean," the mung is mighty for cleansing the body and reestablishing the metabolic Fire. Whenever I am feeling lethargic or toxic from overindulgence, I start soaking mung beans. While even saying the words "mung bean" may give you an immediate vision of Birkenstocks and braids, put your hippie fears aside for a moment. Mung beans are delightfully verdant green when whole, sunny yellow when split. Mung is one of the easiest beans to digest when they are well-spiced and cooked. The old teachings of Ayurveda recommended mung bean soup for the very old and sick. Mung beans are light, full of antioxidants, antiinflammatory, and super nutrient-dense. Mung beans have a slightly sweet and astringent taste. Add some oil or ghee when you cook them, as this helps their nutrients reach the deepest layer of our tissue. Soak whole green mung beans overnight, split mung beans for half an hour. Check out the mung-inspired recipes in Appendix A (pages 243–244) to start tapping into the power of this little bean.

A Word on Almonds

I eat almonds all day in my car and at work. I heard they were healthy!

It depends. Here's why: Almonds are much more beneficial to the body when we eat them in moderation (like 8–10) and remove the skins. Their skins have an acidic and astringent mild cyanide that prevents birds and other critters from eating them. It is actually toxic to the liver, and while it may not kill you, it will definitely kill off some of the goodness within you. Once skinned, the creamy sweet almond is healing for vata in small amounts. Almonds are easiest to digest when they have been soaked for 24–36 hours. I find that women tend to over-use almonds as a meal-replacement for an over-active lifestyle. Even though almonds are healthy, they are not a loving meal.

A Word on Nuts in General

I love nuts and use them as meal replacements!

My response would be, "Are you experiencing gas and bloating?" I find that many busy women snack on nuts as a healthy, energy-packed superfood. In very small amounts, this is okay. But nuts are heavy and drying. As a meal replacement, oily nuts stress the liver and the digestive system. This may be related to their high arginine (an amino acid) content and general heaviness. Therefore, enjoy nuts as a garnish or eat a few on an occasional basis. Also, ask yourself, *Why do I believe I'm not worth a warm nourishing lunch?*

A Word on Raw Foods

I've heard that eating raw food is healthier. Is that true?

It is so tempting to regard raw food as the panacea for good nutrition. When I think of raw food, I think of "the beautiful people." You know: Los Angeles, the beach, tanned skin, toned bodies. Sadly, many of us bought into the myth that raw food will turn us all into glowing Hollywood babes. Ayurveda begs to bust the myth. Ayurvedic practitioner John Joseph Immel puts it really well when he says that "the measure of good food is not just its contents, but its interaction with our body."[2]

While raw, colorful fruits and veggies can offer high amounts of vitamins and nutrients, for most people they are challenging to the digestive system, causing a lot of gas and bloating. Many people turn to raw foods because they feel crappy. They feel crappy because their vital metabolic Fire (agni) is low. But low agni can't digest raw food. So the deal is, no matter how much nutritional benefit raw food offers, if you don't have the digestive Fire to metabolize it, it turns to fermented gut toxins. As Dr. Robert Svoboda, an Ayurvedic expert, points out, "Even the nectar of immortality is a poison if the body can't digest it."[3]

It's a balancing act. Cooked food is easier to digest but cooking does sap some of the good vitamins, minerals, and enzymes out of food. As with most Ayurvedic inquiries, the answer to "Is raw better?" is, "It just depends." If your metabolic Fire is strong and it is summer, then enjoy some raw! If it is winter, you have a vata constitution, and are feeling a little constipated, avoid "raw" like the plague. In general, pitta folks can digest raw foods more easily than other types.

A Word on Gluten Free

I'm allergic to gluten.

It seems everyone is gluten intolerant these days. We ought to stop and ask how all this gluten intolerance happened, seemingly overnight. Perhaps we are experiencing collective dampened digestive power? I don't think simply producing more processed "gluten-free" products will get to the root of the problem. The root is low metabolic Fire. From an Ayurvedic perspective, decades of canned food, processed TV dinners, and bagged, sliced bread have finally caught up with us. Those of us who may be more in tune or sensitive—or just have constitutionally weaker metabolic capacities—are experiencing a revolt from within. This is when we get things like food allergies and intolerances. Don't be disturbed if this is your situation. Flip back to the section on Boosting Metabolic Fire (page 73) to start rebuilding your belly.

A Word on Seedless Watermelons

I love watermelon—but the seeds are such a pain!

Seedless fruits create seedless people. Seeds in humans = ovaries and sperm.

A Word on Kombucha

I don't drink wine, but I love kombucha!

Well, if you've had three kombuchas today, mama, you are not on the cutting edge of the modern health movement—you are drunk! Okay, maybe that's an exaggeration, but kombucha was traditionally

used in small amounts as a medicine, not as a hot-pink soft drink you pick up on your lunch break. Kombucha is a bubbly, fermented drink, sort of like a yeasty sweet tea. Created by fermenting mushrooms, a kombucha culture is actually a symbiotic colony of bacteria and yeast. Consult with a health practitioner to find out if this beverage is a good medicine for you.

A Word on Wine

Me? I use yoga and meditation to deal with stress. Just kidding, I'm on my third glass of wine tonight.

First, the good news: Aged wine, taken in moderation with food, was used in ancient Ayurveda to boost the digestive Fire. It was recommended in very moderate quantities (enough to fill a large shot glass), and was taken only when someone felt healthy and not depressed. Let me repeat that. Wine is a *depressant*. If you drink it because you are stressed and sad, it may take the edge off those feelings, but it will ultimately lead to more depression. When we use alcohol of any kind habitually and to excess, it is said to reduce our ojas (the body's natural immunity and feeling of satisfaction).

Need any more reasons to stay off the pinot noir? How about the results of the One Million Women study, which found that even one glass of wine a day increased a woman's chances of getting any type of cancer?[4] If you are concerned about keeping your heart healthy, drink some açaí berry juice, which is rich in the same antiaging properties. Açaí berries have ten times more antioxidants than wine.[5] I also suggest getting that juicy "wine-relax" feeling in healthier ways. Check out the recipes section of this book for some nourishing, spicy milks that may do just the trick.

Several Words on Milk

Here's the deal with milk. Yeah, I know you say you can't digest it, sister, but hear me out. Traditionally, milk was never pasteurized, homogenized, hormonified, stripped of all good fats, and pumped full of extra vitamin supplements. It makes sense that much of the milk we drink today produces mucus—it is as far removed from the creamy goodness that comes out of Bessie's teat as Wonder Bread is from a loaf of warm sourdough at your local bakery. You see, Ayurveda always encouraged people to slowly boil their milk before drinking it. Based on ancient "good farming" practices, this process killed off bad bacteria and germs. By slowly boiling it, all the good bacteria and enzymes stay in the milk.

What's more, the things that cause milk reactions, mucus, and lactose intolerance are more related to the homogenization process, not the milk itself. Ayurveda, as well as several interesting research efforts, have shown that homogenization is what makes milk fat hard to digest. Check out Ayurvedic practitioner Dr. John Douillard's website at lifespa.com. You can geek out on milk studies and learn exactly how homogenization takes fat molecules in the milk and force-squeezes them into unrecognizable quasi-milk molecules that no amount of cinnamon can help break down. This turns into what Dr. Douillard calls "foreign sludge in the lymph and blood stream, which sticks to channel walls, creates plaque and allergic responses."[6] Whew! Douillard goes on to suggest that we use either raw unpasteurized, non-homogenized milk, or pick up some whipping cream that is non-homogenized and vat pasteurized, and dilute it with water. Check the references section at the back of this book for some great websites on where to get non-homogenized milk products.

Milk is regarded as precious nourishment in ancient Ayurvedic texts. Cooling and balancing, Ayurveda says that milk is one of the purest natural foods for humans. It was used as a potent aphrodisiac and a treatment for depression, cancer, and kidney failure. It was also used to treat the overweight by giving them a sweet, soothing, satisfying meal replacement. With the appropriate spices (see below) and maybe a little coconut oil or ghee, it was used as a dinner replacement for obese people.

Here's how to drink it.

Try to get raw, unpasteurized, non-homogenized milk. If that's not available, at least go organic. Nonorganic dairy products are full of toxins such as antibiotics, growth hormones, and pesticides. Plus, milk is the essence of cows who have been pumped full of the same gnarly stuff. So get organic milk or avoid milk altogether.

What to drink: whole, 2%, or skim? You can totally have whole milk. That is, as long as your digestion is good and you aren't dealing with a big kapha imbalance (such as a mucus-filled head cold). You can especially have whole milk if it is boiled slowly, well-spiced, and taken before bed. You can have even more (especially whole milk) if you are a hardworking woman who feels exhausted but can't fall sleep.

Don't drink milk cold. Boil it slowly and drink it warm. If it feels too heavy for your belly, add some water.

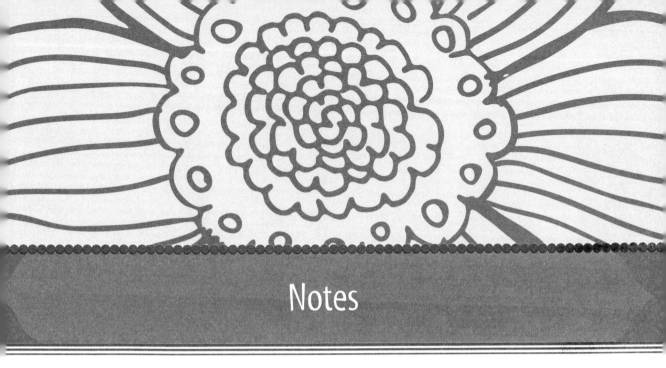

Notes

Introduction

1. Marc Halpern, *Principles of Ayurvedic Medicine* (Nevada City, NV: The California College of Ayurveda, 2007), 17.

2. Domonik Wujastyk, ed., *The Roots of Ayurveda: Selection from Sanskrit Medical Writings* (New York: Penguin Books, 2003).

Chapter One

1. Acharya Vaidya Yadavji Trikamji, ed. and trans., *Charaka Samhita, with Ayurveda-Dipika Commentary of Chakrapanidatta*, fifth edition (Varanasi: Chaukhamba Sanskrit Samsthan, 2001).

2. "Insufficient Sleep Is a Public Health Epidemic," Centers for Disease Control and Prevention, accessed April 2014, http://www.cdc.gov/features/dssleep/; Institute of Medicine, *Sleep Disorders and Sleep Deprivation: An Unmet Public Health Problem* (Washington, DC: The National Academies Press, 2006).

Chapter Two

1. Mark Hyman Rapaport, Pamela Schettler, and Catherine Bresee, "A Preliminary Study of the Effects of a Single Session of Swedish Massage on Hypothalamic-Pituitary-Adrenal and Immune Function in Normal Individuals," *Journal of Alternative and Complementary Medicine* (September 2010), http://www.ncbi.nlm.nih.gov/pmc/articles/PMC3107905/.

Chapter Four

1. Lori Gaspar, "Dr. David Frawley: Reuniting Yoga and Ayurveda," *YOGA Chicago* (July–August 2004), http://yogachicago.com/2014/03/dr-david-frawley-reuniting-yoga-and-ayurveda/.

Chapter Six

1. Vasant Lad and Usha Lad, *Ayurvedic Cooking for Self-Healing* (Albuquerque, NM: Ayurvedic Press, 1997).

Chapter Seven

1. David Frawley and Vasant Lad, *The Yoga of Herbs: An Ayurvedic Guide to Herbal Medicine* (Twin Lakes, MN: Lotus Press, 1986), 25–33; Pratima Raichur, *Absolute Beauty: Radiant Skin and Inner Harmony Through the Ancient Secrets of Ayurveda* (New York: HarperPerennial, 1999), 389.

Chapter Eight

1. Dalai Lama, "Western Women Can Come to the Rescue of the World," posted by Victor Chan (January 2010), http://dalailamacenter.org/blog-post/western-women-can-come-rescue-world.

2. Nicole Daedone, "Orgasm: The Cure for Hunger in the Western Woman," TEDxSF, http://www.youtube.com/watch?v=s9QVq0EM6g4.

3. Kermit Baker, "Kitchens and Baths Benefit from Broader Housing Recovery, Feature New Functions and Activities," *The American Institute of Architects*, http://www.aia.org/practicing/AIAB097963.

Chapter Nine

1. Robert E. Svoboda, *Prakriti: Your Ayurvedic Constitution* (Detroit, MI: Lotus Press, 1998), 118.

2. "Annual Sleep in America Poll Exploring Connections with Communications Technology Use and Sleep," NationalSleepFoundation.org, March 7, 2011, http://sleepfoundation.org/media-center/press-release/annual-sleep-america-poll-exploring-connections-communications-technology-use-.

3. Claudia Welch, *Balance Your Hormones, Balance Your Life: Achieving Optimal Health and Wellness through Ayurveda, Chinese Medicine, and Western Science* (New York: Da Capo Lifelong Books, 2011).

4. Ibid.

5. Cosmetic Ingredient Review Panel, Washington, DC, "Ingredients Found Unsafe for Use in Cosmetics." Environmental Working Group (February 2012), http://www.cir-safety .org/sites/default/files/U-unsafe%202-02-2012%20final.pdf.

6. Working Group on Endocrine Disrupters of the Scientific Committee on Toxicity, Ecotoxicity and the Environment (CSTEE) of DG XXIV, Consumer Policy and Consumer Health Protection, "CSTEE Opinion on Human and Wildlife Health Effects of Endocrine Disrupting Chemicals, with Emphasis on Wildlife and on Ecotoxicology Test Methods" (March 1999), http://ec.europa.eu/health/archive/ph_risk/committees/sct /documents/out37_en.pdf.

7. Raichur, *Absolute Beauty*.

8. Varsha Chaudhari, Manjusha Rajagopala, Sejal Mistry, and D. B. Vaghela, "Role of *Pradhamana Nasya* and *Trayodashanga Kwatha* in the Management of *Dushta Pratishyaya* with Special Reference to Chronic Sinusitis," *Ayu* 31, 3 (July–September 2010): 325–331, http://www.ncbi.nlm.nih.gov/pmc/articles/PMC3221066/.

9. Abhinav Singh and Bharathi Purohit, "Tooth Brushing, Oil Pulling, and Tissue Regeneration: A Review of Holistic Approaches to Oral Health," *Journal of Ayurveda and Integrative Medicine* 2, no. 2 (April-June 2011): 64–68.

10. S. Asokan, J. Rathan, M. S. Muthu, P. V. Rathna, P. Emmadi, Raghuraman, and Chamundeswari, "Effect of Oil Pulling on *Streptococcus Mutans* Count in Plaque and Saliva Using Dentocult Sm Strip Mutans Test: A Randomized, Controlled, Triple-Blind Study," *Journal of Indian Society of Pedodontics and Preventive Dentistry* 26, no. 1 (March 2008): 12–17, http://www.ncbi.nlm.nih.gov/pubmed/18408265.

11. T. Durai Anand, C. Pothiraj, R. M. Gopinath, and B. Kayalvizhi, "Effect of Oil-Pulling on Dental Caries Causing Bacteria," *African Journal of Microbiology Research* 2, no. 3 (March 2008): 63–66; H. V. Amith, Anil V. Ankola, L. Nagesh, "Effect of Oil Pulling on Plaque and Gingivitis," *Journal of Oral Health and Community Dentistry* 1, no. 1 (January 2007): 12–18.

12. John Douillard, "The Truth About Oil Pulling," LifeSpa, http://lifespa.com/the-truth -about-oil-pulling/.

Chapter 10

1. V. Morhenn, L. E. Beavin, and P. J. Zak, "Massage Increases Oxytocin and Reduces Adrenocorticotropin Hormone in Humans," *Journal of Alternative Therapies in Health and Medicine* 18, no. 6 (November–December 2012): 11–18, http://www.ncbi.nlm.nih.gov /pubmed/23251939.

Chapter 11

1. A. Blumenthal, M. A. Babyak, K. A. Moore, W. E. Craighead, S. Herman, P. Khatri, R. Waugh, et al, "Effects of Exercise Training on Older Patients with Major Depression," *Archives of Internal Medicine* 159, no. 19 (October 1999): 2349–2356, http://www.ncbi .nlm.nih.gov/pubmed/10547175.

Chapter 12

1. Marci Shimoff, *Happy for No Reason: 7 Steps to Being Happy from the Inside Out* (New York: Simon & Schuster, 2008); University of Wisconsin-Madison, "University of Wisconsin Study Reports Sustained Changes in Brain and Immune Function After Meditation," *Science-Daily* (February 4, 2003), www.sciencedaily.com/releases /2003/02/030204074125.htm; Susan Kuchinskas, "Meditation Boosts Mood, Immune System," WebMD (February 2009), http://www.webmd.com/mental-health/features/meditation-heals-body-and-mind.

2. Kevin Chen, C. C. Berger, E. Manheimer, D. Forde, J. Magidson, L. Dachman, and C. W. Lejuez, "Meditative Therapies for Reducing Anxiety: A Systematic Review and Meta-Analysis of Randomized Controlled Trials," *Depression and Anxiety* 29, no. 7 (July 2012): 1–18.

3. Rolf Sovik, *Moving Inward: The Journey to Meditation* (Honesdale, PA: Himalayan Institute Press, 2007), 14.

4. Phonetic translation by Christopher Wallis.

5. Ibid.

Chapter 13

1. Vinod Verma, *The Kamasutra for Women: The Modern Woman's Way to Sensual Fulfillment and Health* (New York: Kodansha, 1997).

2. Nicholas Carr, "Author Nicholas Carr: The Web Shatters Focus, Rewires Brains," *Wired* magazine (May 2010), http://www.wired.com/2010/05/ff_nicholas_carr/2/.

3. Alan Hirsch, *What Flavor Is Your Personality? Discover Who You Are by Looking at What You Eat* (Naperville, IL: Sourcebooks, 2001); L. A. Johnson, "Sexy Scents: The Nose Knows the Best Sensory Stimuli," Post-Gazette.com (February 2001), http://old.post-gazette.com /magazine/20010214scentoflove2.asp.

Chapter 14

1. Cassandra Lorius, *101 Nights of Tantric Sex: How to Make Each Night a New Way of Sexual Ecstasy* (New York: Barnes and Noble, 2007), 58.

2. Shiva Rea, *Tending the Heart Fire: Living in Flow with the Pulse of Life* (Louisville, CO: Sounds True, 2014), 110.

3. Tom Kenyon and Judi Sion, *The Magdalen Manuscript: The Alchemies of Horus & the Sex Magic of Isis* (Ashland, OR: Tom Kenyon Orb, 2006).

4. Anil Ananthaswamy, "Hormones Converge for Couples in Love," *New Scientist Online* (May 2004), http://www.newscientist.com/article/dn4957-hormones-converge-for-couples -in-love.html#.U0q8Oxa81UQ.

5. Ellen Berscheid and Pamela Regan, *The Psychology of Interpersonal Relationships* (Mahwah, NJ: Prentice-Hall, 2005).

Chapter 16

1. Verma, *The Kamasutra for Women*.

2. Margie Profet, "Menstruation as a Defense against Pathogens Transported by Sperm," *The Quarterly Review of Biology* 68, no. 3 (September 1993): 335–386, doi:10.1086/418170.

3. U.S. Department of Health and Human Services, Office on Women's Health, "Pre-menstrual Syndrome (PMS) fact sheet," http://www.womenshealth.gov/publications/ our-publications/fact-sheet/premenstrual-syndrome.pdf.

4. Eckart Tolle, *A New Earth: Awakening to Your Life's Purpose* (New York: Penguin, 2008), 142.

5. Judith Orloff, "The Health Benefits of Tears," adapted from *Emotional Freedom: Liberate Yourself from Negative Emotions and Transform Your Life* (New York: Three Rivers Press, 2011), 194, www.drjudithorloff.com/Free-Articles/The-Health-Benefits-of-Tears-copy.htm.

6. Jane Bennett and Alexandra Pope, *The Pill: Are You Sure It's for You?* (Crows Nest, New South Wales, Australia: Allen & Unwin, 2008), 52–53.

7. Welch, *Balance Your Hormones, Balance Your Life*.

Appendix B

1. Welch, *Balance Your Hormones, Balance Your Life*.

2. Vasant Lad, *The Complete Book of Ayurvedic Home Remedies* (New York: Harmony Books, 1999).

Appendix C

1. A. Trichopoulou and P. Lagiou, "Worldwide Patterns of Dietary Lipids Intake and Health Implications," *American Journal of Clinical Nutrition* 66 (October 1997).

2. John Joseph Immel, "The Raw Versus Cooked Food Debate," *Joyful Belly*, http://www.joyfulbelly.com/Ayurveda/article/The-Raw-Versus-Cooked-Food-Debate/269.

3. Ibid.

4. "Million Women Study Shows Even Moderate Alcohol Consumption Associated with Increased Cancer Risk," *Journal of the National Cancer Institute* 101, no. 5 (2009), http://jnci.oxfordjournals.org/content/101/5/281.2.full.

5. Ashley Cox, "Açaí Berries: Super Food or Hype?" *Science 2.0* (October 2008), http://www.science20.com/variety_tap/acai_berries_super_food_or_hype.

6. John Douillard, "Stop Eating Dairy until You Read This Report!" LifeSpa (November 2010), http://lifespa.com/stop-eating-dairy-until-you-read-this-report/.

Resources

Katie Silcox Yoga Retreats, Training Events, and Education

Katie's website, www.katiesilcoxyoga.com, includes Katie's speaking events, yoga teacher trainings and workshops, luscious self-care retreats, and women's holistic healing events. It also includes more information, including videos, resources, recipes, and online courses in the field of Tantra and Ayurveda.

Katie's blog on all-things Tantra and Ayurveda: www.parayogini.com.

Check out the complete *Healthy Happy Sexy* website for audio recordings of meditations and yoga nidra, plus special offers, recipes, and online events and courses: www.healthyhappysexylife.com.

Herbal Resources

Mountain Rose Herbs www.mountainroseherbs.com
Starwest Botanicals www.starwest-botanicals.com
Organic India www.organicindia.com

Pacific Botanicals www.pacificbotanicals.com
Trinity Ava Herbalism trinityava.com

Herbs, Oils, Neti Pots, Tongue Scrapers, Education, and Chyawanprash

Banyan Botanicals www.banyanbotanicals.com
Himalayan Institute www.himalayaninstitute.org

My All-Time Favorite Ayurveda Body-Care Line and Bodywork Heaven

Earthbody Sacred Skincare, San Francisco
  earthbodyskincare.com

Other Great Body-Care Lines

Aromabliss aromabliss.com/Daily.htm
Śarada Ayurveda www.saradausa.com
Bindi www.bindi.com
Qori Inti Amazonian Herbals www.qoriintiherbals.com/shop
Rupam's Apothecary www.rupamherbals.com
Kama Ayurveda at Pure Natural purenatural.ew.store
Loving Hands Ayurveda lovinghandsayurveda.com
Trillium Organics www.trilliumorganics.com
Chagrin Valley Soap & Salve Company
  www.chagrinvalleysoapandsalve.com
Auromere (toothpaste) www.auromere.com
TheraNeem (toothpaste) organixsouth.com/theraneem.html

Essential Oils

Floracopeia www.floracopeia.com
Essential Aura www.essentialaura.com

Original Swiss Aromatics www.originalswissaromatics.com
Veriditas botanicals www.veriditasbotanicals.com

Ayurvedic Education Institutions

The Ayurvedic Institute www.ayurveda.com
The California College of Ayurveda www.ayurvedacollege.com
Mount Madonna Center www.mountmadonna.org
The Pacific Center of Ayurveda
   www.pacificcenterofayurveda.com
American Institute of Vedic Studies www.vedanet.com

Tantric Hatha Yoga Education

ParaYoga www.parayoga.com

Recommended Reading

Balance Your Hormones, Balance Your Life by Dr. Claudia Welch
Any books by Dr. Vasant Lad
Any books by Dr. Robert Svoboda
Any books by David Frawley
Any books by Maya Tiwari
The Kamasutra for Women by Vinod Verma
The Four Desires by Rod Stryker
Healing Your Life: Lessons on the Path of Ayurveda by
   Dr. Marc Halpern

Cookbooks and Resources for Ayurvedic Cooking

Eat, Taste, Heal by Thomas Yarema, Daniel Rhoda, and
   Johnny Brannigan
Ayurvedic Cooking for Self-Healing by Usha Lad and Vasant Lad

Ayurvedic Cooking for Westerners by Amadea Morningstar

Heaven's Banquet: Vegetarian Cooking for Lifelong Health the Ayurveda Way by Miriam Kasin Hospodar

Joyful Belly www.joyfulbelly.com (best Ayurveda-inspired website!)

Ayurveda-Friendly Menstrual Products

The Diva Cup divacup.com

The Moon Cup www.mooncup.com

Organic tampons www.seventhgeneration.com and
www.natracare.com

Jade Eggs

Jade Eggs www.jadeeggs.com

Chinese Secret www.chinese-secret.com

TantraNova www.tantranova.com

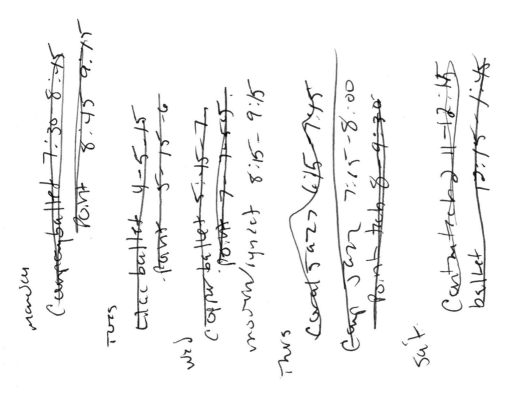